A RECONSTRUCTION OF THE SENSORY WORLD OF AUTISM

Olga Bogdashina

Olga Bogdashina

Sheffield Hallam University Press
Learning Centre
City Campus
Pond Street
Sheffield S1 1WB

First published 2001

Designed and typeset by Design Studio, Learning Centre, Sheffield Hallam University

 ISBN 0 86339 930 4

Sheffield Hallam University

Sheffield **H**allam **A**utism **R**esource **E**xchange: autism - a series

Series editor: Nick Hodge, Senior Lecturer in Autism at Sheffield Hallam University and Director of SHARE.

All of the works which appear in this series have one aspect in common; autism.

They may be: text or video, theoretical or practical, substantial or brief and yet all will contain information of use to those who are autistic or family and friends of autistic people or the professionals who work in collaboration with them.

The range of works within this series will be varied and colourful. In discussing the topic of autism, how could it be anything less.

Series editor's preface.

It is especially pleasing to launch this series, 'SHARE: autism - a series', with a work by Olga Bogdashina as she writes not only as an academic but also as a parent of a young autistic man.

This work focuses on an area of research, which has been largely neglected to date, that of the sensory impact of autism. As a teacher of autistic pupils I was often aware that autism might well have affected the sensory perceptions of the pupils I worked with but felt that I rarely modified what I was doing to take account of this. I was often left pondering questions such as; should I open or close blinds, speak louder or more quietly, insist on pupils looking at me when I speak or allow them only to listen, make my classroom a visual delight or keep it understated? I had no means of assessing how each individual was experiencing the environment and so worked only on instinct.

Structured observation is essential if we are to make any attempt to understand how the world might appear to an autistic person. The checklist contained within this book is an excellent starting point for guiding our focus, helping us to build a truer picture of a particular person's perspective. We cannot expect all the work to come from those who are autistic. We too must learn to empathise and see the world from other viewpoints.

I would have found useful also the comprehensive account, within this text, of the sensory experiences recorded by autistic people. This would have helped me in my understanding and made me more sensitive to the needs of my pupils. It would also have offered comfort to those pupils who perceive themselves as "different", to know that there are others who also experience the world in these "different" ways.

More research is needed in this field. Especially research such as this, which results in practical application. Olga's contribution to this area of study is indeed both valuable and timely.

Nick Hodge

About the Author

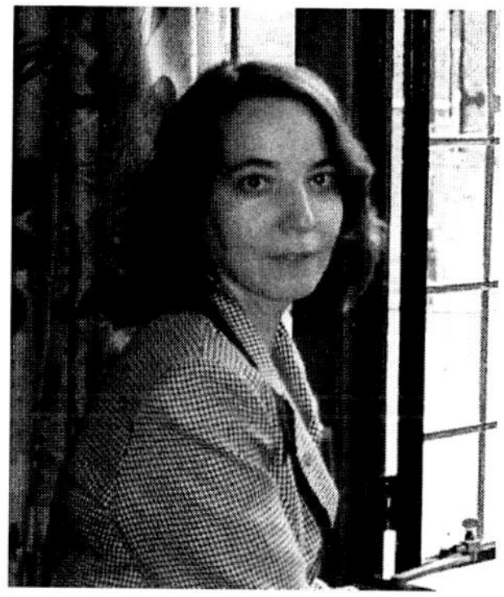

Professor Olga Bogdashina was born in Krasnoyarsk, Siberia; educated at Moscow University (Linguistics) and for 11 years lived in Gorlovka in Ukraine where she was a Principal Lecturer and head of the Department at the State Teacher Training Institute of Foreign Languages. Olga's son, aged 12, is autistic. Autism has limited recognition in the countries of the former USSR. In 1994 Olga established and became President of the first Autism Society in Ukraine – "From Despair to Hope". She is Director of a voluntary day school in Gorlovka for children on the autism spectrum. Olga has had several articles, leaflets and a book "Autism: Definitions and Diagnoses" published in Ukraine and several articles in professional journals in Belgium and France.

Dedicated to my son who inspired me to write it.

Olga Bogdashina

Contents

Olga Bogdashina

INTRODUCTION

Since the first identification of autism in 1943 (Kanner) a lot of research has been carried out to study this condition from different perspectives. What has not been taken into account by the experts in the field, however, is the opinion of the 'native experts' – autistic individuals themselves. Despite the fact that many people with autism have tried to communicate their views and insights, these attempts have mostly passed without much professional notice, one of the reasons being, their views and insights are unconventional to the majority of people (so-called 'normal' people).

Here we try to show that 'different' does not mean 'abnormal' or 'defective', and 'normalcy' is a very relative term, as the 'norm' is often applied to the performance of majority, and it is more justifiable to term it 'typical'. To avoid having to use the term 'normal', autistic people at Autism Network International (ANI, founded by Jim Sinclair and Donna Williams in 1992) have introduced a new term – 'Neurologically Typical' (NT) to describe non-autistic people.

Here I deliberately use more often the term autistic people rather than people with autism, because autism is not something that is just attached to them and can be removed. I am aware about the 'people first and than disability' approach, however, without autism they would be different people as being autistic means being different. If people with autism themselves prefer to name themselves autistic why should we be so shy to call them that? Just to show them our respect? But there are other ways to do it. Why should we be ashamed of calling them autistic? Autism is not something to be ashamed of.

For autistic people, autism is a way of being. It is pervasive, it colours every experience, every sensation, perception, thought, emotion, in sort, every aspect of existence (Sinclair, 1993). They do not respond in a way we expect them to, because they have different systems of perception and communication. Bob Morris (1999) calls it a different set of SPATS – Senses, Perceptions, Abilities and Thinking Systems, that are not in the same spectral ranges as NT individuals. Of course, it is very difficult to communicate with someone who uses a different 'language' (and autistic people are 'foreigners' in any culture). But it is equally wrong to use non-autistic methods to teach and treat autistic children. It is sure to fail and sometimes even to damage their life.

We have to give up our conventional non-autistic assumptions and let them teach us of their communication systems in order to build bridges between the two worlds. We follow Donna Williams's recommendation of the way to help people with autism: "If you have a camel which is finding it hard to walk under the weight of all the straws on its back, the easiest way to make it easier for the camel to walk is to take as many straws off its back as possible"... and not to train "the camel to walk or appear to walk whilst carrying the straws. To take the straws off the camel's back, you have to do two things. One is to identify them and second is to know how to remove them." (1996, 87).

At present as there are no known medical tests to indicate autism, the diagnosis is based on the presence of the specific behaviours (DSM-IV, ICD-10), viz. impairments of social interaction, communication and imagination, known collectively as the Triad of Impairments (Wing, 1992). However, these behaviours are seen as a cluster of purposeful compensatory reactions caused by some fundamental impairment(s) and cannot be considered as primary characteristics. It is no use trying to eliminate these behaviours without identifying underlying causes, no matter how much these behaviours interfere with the teaching or treatment of autistic children.

Since Kanner's identification of autism (1943) different theories of the probable deficits in autism have emerged. Since the 1970s the main emphasis has been made on the cognitive development of autistic children; different theories of cognitive deficits have been originated: "theory of mind" (Baron-Cohen et al., 1985), central coherence theory (Frith, 1989), executive functioning deficit theory (Ozonoff, 1995), and some others. All these theories suggest that low-level perceptual processes are intact in autism and information processing up to the point of interpretation by a central system can be assumed to be normal in autism (Frith, 1989).

Although in the 1960s-70s the idea of possible sensory-perceptual abnormalities as one of the core features of the disorder was put forward (Rimland, 1964) and theory of sensory dysfunction was formulated (Delacato, 1974) until recently it has been ignored by the researchers.

What makes one wonder, is that, though unusual sensory experiences have been observed in autistic people for many years and are confirmed by personal accounts of high-functioning autistic individuals, it is still listed as an associated but not essential feature of autism in the main diagnostic classifications – DSM-IV (APA, 1994) and ICD-10 (WHO, 1992).

At present it is commonly recognised that there are many possible causes of autism and some researchers (Waterhouse, 2000) distinguish several types of autism ("autisms") all of which result in the same behavioural patterns (impairments of social interaction, communication and imagination). Though many different problems can produce similar symptoms, what makes it autism is a specific combination of these problems reflected in the Triad of impairments. There is a scientific evidence that deficits in information processing that is both perceptive and executive, is found in all persons within the autistic spectrum, though the role of sensory-perceptual problems is still very controversial.

The analysis of the personal accounts of autistic people shows that autism is largely a condition relating to sensory processing, though the current diagnostic systems blindly ignore the fact. Temple Grandin (1996a) suggests that there is a continuum of sensory processing problems for most autistic people, which goes from fractured disjointed images at one end to a slight abnormality at the other.

This work attempts to reconstruct the sensory world of autism in order to help professionals and parents understand the way autistic people experience the world, as often very well-meaning specialists are "failing people with autism… (and) most (autistic people) have not been helped at all, many have felt degraded and some have been harmed" (Gerland, 1998) because of the misunderstanding and misinterpretation of the condition. This is the attempt to describe possible sensory experiences (not always necessarily abnormalities) based on the personal accounts of autistic people. If we can understand the causes of certain behaviours we can accept these behaviours. If we know what to look for, it will be easier for us to understand the person's problems and abilities and to find appropriate methods to identify and remove the 'straws'. Moreover, understanding of the way autistic people experience the world will bring respect to people with autism in their attempts to survive and live a productive life in our world instead of unacceptance often exhibited by the general public.

What lacks in most studies on the sensory dysfunction in autism is the opinion and views on the problem of the autistic people themselves. Bob Morris (1999) calls it 'the original error' of the investigations, i.e. trying to reconstruct the 'autistic world' using methods and perceptions of non-autistics. To avoid this error the personal accounts of autistic individuals were seen as the main source of information about this condition. As Donna Williams (2000) states, "if you want to understand French you get a native French speaker, if you want to understand Autistic, you approach an Autistic person". The texts for analysis included books and articles written by autistic individuals. These were supplemented with talks at conferences and personal communication with high-functioning autistic individuals.

To avoid repetition, the 'autistic status' of the authors is not specified. A list of the key authors and their works is given in References. During the analysis of the personal accounts it was decided to replace the term 'types of sensory dysfunction' by the term 'types of sensory experiences', as not all the experiences turned out to be 'dysfunctional' or 'defective' but rather 'different' or 'showing superability' (e.g., synaesthesia, 'resonance', 'daydreaming', 'acute vision/hearing' etc.) and might be considered as strengths rather than deficits.

Before we discuss the possible patterns of sensory experiences in autism it is necessary to give a brief explanation of why the role of these differences should not be ignored. This can be found in chapter 1. In the next chapter the possible sensory experiences classified into 20 categories are described. These are by no means a complete set of the descriptors. Further research (and co-operation with autistic individuals) is needed. However, I feel, it would be a good start to achieving an understanding of a sensory world of autism.

Each descriptor is followed by a 'what to look for' section, to help with the identification of this particular characteristic with the 'behaviours on the surface'. Sometimes we cannot explain the behaviour because we don't know what might cause it. I hope the descriptions of the behaviours will help find the answers to some 'why does he do this' questions.

While reading the descriptions and especially explanations and experiences given by the autistic authors, I'd advise the reader to do two things: 1. Try to simulate these autistic sensory experiences in order to imagine at least what it could be like for them. 2. Think of any autistic person you have known. Is it about him/her? Does his behaviour make sense now?

After 'exploration' of the sensory world we move to the 'rainbows' – special graphs that will help identify possible different experiences of each child in order to work with him 'on his territory'.

At the end of the book one can find the case studies of autistic children whose 'rainbows' show that despite the same diagnosis their perceptions are different, and our approaches to each of them should take into account their differences.

Chapter 1

SENSORY DYSFUNCTION OR DIFFERENT SENSORY EXPERIENCES?

In recent decades there have appeared different conceptions of autism which highlight sensory-perceptual abnormalities as the basis of core features of the disorder and that all symptoms of autism are simply a consequence of the brain injury that makes brains of autistic children perceive inputs from the world differently from non-injured brains. Autism is sometimes defined as sensory dysfunction (Delacato, 1974), a sensory integrative disorder in which the brain is not able to attach meaning to sensations and organise them into percepts and finally into concepts (Ayres, 1979), etc.

Unusual sensory experience that is not considered as a diagnostic characteristic in the main diagnostic classifications of autism is claimed by some authors to be a primary characteristic feature that is able to account for the basic symptoms of autism which are considered to be essential according to DSM-IV and ICD-10. Thus, abnormal perceptions might give rise to high levels of anxiety, this, in turn, results in the obsessive or compulsive behaviours, thus making the more commonly accepted criteria, in fact, secondary developmental problems (Delacato, 1974).

The indirect evidence that these assumptions might be true comes from the research in the fields of sensory deprivation and visual and/or auditory impairments. Sensory deprivation studies (Doman, 1984) show that sudden and nearly complete deprivation of stimulation through the five senses can lead to autistic-like behaviours (withdrawal, stereotyped movements, etc.), but these problems are reversible with proper stimulation. The symptoms of sensory deprivation in animals and many autistic symptoms are similar as well: animals confined to a barren environment are excitable and engage in stereotyped behaviours, self-injury (Grandin, 1996b).

The recent research (Cass, 1996) has shown that some similar behaviours occur in children who are blind and in those who are autistic: impairments in social interaction, communication, stereotyped movements. Gense and Gense (1994) have shown the many ways in which the behaviour of children with autism and those who have visual impairments is similar, for example, such behaviours as rocking and rhythmic head banging, spinning objects, or perimeter hugging (especially in large spaces) and needing to touch everything in a room before settling down. Concerning autism, this is often considered as obsessional ritual behaviour without explaining a functional base to this behaviour. Autistic people argue that the original cause of it is of a perceptual nature. Donna Williams, for example, when asked why she does this, says that she has difficulty perceiving herself in relation to her environment until she has done this; it gives her security by helping interpret her environment. Thus, the following characteristics (Cass, 1996) might be "normal" for blind children: absence of eye contact, referential eye gaze and pointing; repetitive behaviours; language abnormalities; orientating behaviours (e.g., smelling, touching objects, etc.). There arises a question: are autistic children "blind" in a way, i.e. have they got a sort of distorted perception?

There have been also observed common features in the language development of children with autism and those with visual impairments, for example, echolalia and pronoun reversal – distinctive features of 'autistic language' – are also observed in the language of children with visual impairments (Fay & Schuler, 1980). It is recognised that there is a critical role for visual stimulation for the development of communication.

The similar 'autistic' characteristics are observed in deaf children, though in a less degree. The possible explanation for this lies in the fact that around 75-80% of the information about the world comes through vision, so a blind child has to make sense of or process a very different set of sensory information that may develop emotional and psychological problems and result in 'autistic' behaviour. The researchers (Cass, 1996) assume that the autistic-like picture observed in a proportion of blind children arises from the same core deficit as that in sighted autistic children.

Though blindness means there is an absence of visual information about the world, it affects all levels of functioning. To draw a parallel one might assume autism means there are distortions of visual/auditory/gustatory/olfactory/tactile information about the world. Whereas the blind/the deaf/the deaf-blind have other senses, which work properly, to compensate their vision or hearing, and 'see' through their ears, nose and hands, or 'hear' through their hands and eyes, autistic people often cannot rely on their senses as all of them might be affected in some way.

There exist several standardised instruments for evaluating sensory integrative dysfunction, e.g., the Sensory Integration and Praxis Tests for children aged 4 to 8 (Ayres, 1989), the DeGangi-Berk Test of Sensory Integration for children aged 3 to 5 (Berk & DeGangi, 1983), but these tests do not assess the child in natural settings ('office tests') and are aimed only at identifying deficits. Besides, the age limit does not allow the assessment of the trends of sensory development and compensatory strategies acquired by the individual.

In the Geneva Centre for Autism (Walker & Cantello, 1994) a survey was conducted to gain more insights into sensory experiences of autistic people: through the Internet autistic people were asked to complete the survey anonymously. According to the data obtained, 81% of respondents reported differences in visual perception, 87% - in hearing, 77% - in tactile perception, 30% - in taste, and 56% - in smell.

All these data give some evidence of possible role of distorted sensory perception in autism.

Although recently there have appeared a number of works highlighting perceptual abnormalities in autism, to date, these possible abnormalities and their role in causing autistic behaviours have not been systematically investigated. More research work is needed to find out whether perceptual problems are core features in the fundamental impairment(s) in the autistic condition, which senses are affected, the intensity the senses work, etc.

During the analysis of the personal accounts of autistic individuals the main questions "asked" were: how do they see their difference; what do they think their main problems are; what role does sensory perception play in autism, if any; and what are their sensory experiences?

Most of the autistic authors emphasise that they report about his/her own experiences, and only a few, who have conducted their own research, claim that they speak on behalf of the others (e.g., Morris, 1999). As autism is a spectrum disorder and the symptoms vary from mild to severe ones, it was expected that there would be many variations in the answers. However, although the experiences described are very individual, it has turned out that the main points are very similar.

They did understand that they were different already in early life, but they did not know why. It is no wonder that they are often unaware they perceive the world differently because they have nothing else to compare their perception with. Bob Morris explains: "if you are born with different perceptions, you have no way of knowing your individual perceptions are not the same as the other 99% of the population, until your differences are called to your attention" (1999). The first realisation of the nature of their differences comes in late teens or even later (Lawson, 1998; Willey, 1999; Williams, 1992). For example, it took Liane Willey many years before she realised that she did and thought many things that others did not; she saw how peculiar her world was – not wrong or embarrassing or unessential – just different.

The personal accounts reveal that one of the main problems they experience is their abnormal perception (Gerland, 1997; Grandin, 1986; 1996a,b; Lawson, 1998; O'Neill, 1999; Willey, 1999; Williams, 1992; and others). For example, J.G.T.VanDalen believes that the true invisible deep-rooted cause of all social and emotional problems is of a perceptual nature, and autism to be really understood, has to be seen above all as a perceptual deficit (1995, 11). Temple Grandin states that some episodes of difficult behaviour were directly caused by sensory difficulties (1986; 1996). For Donna Williams her expressive difficulties were secondary and sprang from the primary inconsistencies in her perception of the world around her (1992; 1996; 1998). Bob Morris (1999) argues that autistic people have a different set of SPATS – Senses, Perceptions, Abilities and

Thinking Systems, that are not in the same ranges as non-autistic people. In his opinion, the main problem is in misunderstanding of the condition.

To illustrate the idea of misidentification and misunderstanding of autistic people by NT individuals Bob Morris (1999) uses Hans Andersen's story "The Ugly Duckling": A swan egg became misplaced into a duck's nest. As it grew, it was seen as a poor performing odd duck. But in time, and after correct identification, the swan was shown to be physically more stately, majestic, and powerful than any duck could even hope to be. To describe people with autism ("swans") Morris uses the term Neurologically Cygnus (NC), from the Latin word 'cygnus', which means 'swan'. The author concludes that if we recognise that we have complementary, weak and strong capability patterns in our respective SPATS, the NC person can have life, not life-support, for life. Morris's advice to professionals is to include SPATS in the diagnosis checklist and to teach the all-wise ducks how to recognise, handle and develop a swan, instead of trying to mould the swan into a defective duck.

Many autistic authors emphasize that there are beneficial "side-effects" of autism that could far outweigh the negatives (Kochmeister; Grandin; O'Neill; Sinclair).

The fact that autistic people do share common systems of perception and thinking is confirmed by many autistic individuals: they report that they have very few problems communicating with and understanding people 'of their own kind' (Dekker, Williams). Though there are plenty of varieties in their perception, in general autistic people are no more all different than non-autistics when SPATS are considered as a whole (Morris, 1999).

The analysis of the personal accounts confirmed that autism is largely a condition relating to sensory processing. As the systems work differently their responses to sensory stimuli are 'normal', from an autistic point of view, though different and unconventional, and not abnormal or defective.

It seems wrong to use non-autistic methods to teach and treat autistic children. There are always two ways to look at things: the non-autistic way and the autistic way (Bovee). This analysis was designed to reveal the second way.

There is a traditional description of an autistic person as "living in a world of his own". But I would distinguish not two "worlds": "theirs" – "autistic" and "ours – non-autistic" but three: 1) "theirs – autistic", 2) " a sensory (visual/auditory/tactual/gustatory/olfactory) distorted (different?) world perceived by autistic people" and 3) "ours – non-autistic world" (Bogdashina, 1999). The second 'sensory' world is very different for each individual and reflects the ways their senses work.

In the next chapter an attempt is made to describe and classify possible sensory experiences, which are not always abnormalities, based on the personal accounts of autistic people and close observation of autistic children.

Chapter 2

POSSIBLE PATTERNS OF SENSORY EXPERIENCES IN AUTISM

1. Intensity of the senses (hyper-, hypo-)

Carl Delacato (1974) classified each sensory channel as being

- *Hyper-:* the channel is too open, as a result too much stimulation sets in for the brain to handle;
- *Hypo-:* the channel is not open enough, as a result too little of the stimulation gets in and the brain is deprived;
- *"White noise":* the channel creates its own stimulus because of its faulty operation and, as a result the message from the outside world is overcome by the noise within the system.

Delacato (1974) stated that each sensory channel can be affected in a different way, e.g., a child could be hypovisual, "white noise" auditory, hypo to tastes and smells and hypertactile.

While recognising the revolutionary contribution to the understanding of autism made by Delacato, it seems necessary to argue one point in his theory. Delacato considered that a channel could either be hyper-, hypo-, or "white noise". According to personal accounts of the sufferers themselves, however, it turns out that often one and the same person could experience sensory inputs of one and the same channel at different times from all the three Delacato's categories – hyper-, hypo-, "white noise", - because the intensity with which the channel works often fluctuates. For example, Donna Williams could watch "spots" and "stars" (small particles in the air), showed great discomfort at the bright lights (characteristics of being hypervisual), while she often inspected the objects and things by hand, liked mirrors (hypovisual) and had large pupils, often looked through people and things, disliked eye contact and had distorted visual experience ("white noise").

While describing their unusual sensory experiences autistic individuals prefer the term "hypersensitivity". This term is very broad. In this paper "hypersensitivity" means acute or heightened, or excessive sensitivity; "hyposensitivity" is for below normal sensitivity. Here the terms are deliberately narrowed, as it seems more justifiable to distinguish between different sensory experiences, often conventionally covered by these terms. Below are some examples of hyper- and hyposensitivities of all the channels described by autistic individuals.

Hypersensitivity

Hypervision (seeing "invisible") means that they can see more than other people, i.e. their vision is too acute. For example, as a child, Donna Williams "discovered the air was full of spots", later she learnt that "they are actually air particles" yet her "vision was so hypersensitive that they often became a hypnotic background with the rest of the 'world' fading away" (Williams, 1992, 2, 9).

Annabel Stehli (1991) described her autistic daughter Georgiana who saw "too well" and everything she saw was magnified; "she saw like an eagle"; she saw, for example, every strand of hair "like spaghetti...(that) must have been why she'd been so fascinated by people's hair" (p. 186).

Jasmine O'Neill (1999) describes an autistic person as the person who sees what is around him with extra-acute sight.

Hyperhearing (hearing "inaudible"):

> *"...it was found that my hearing was better than average, and I was able to hear some frequencies that only animals normally hear" (Williams, 1992, 40)*
>
> *"In many ways, I felt my sensory perception was superior to that of my peers. I had the ability to hear noise before they did, which meant that I could tell when the school bus was approaching before others could hear*

> *it. Noises seemed so much louder to me, and I had to move away from conversation at times because the noise hurt my ears"(Lawson, 1998, 30).*
>
> *"My hearing is like having a sound amplifier set on maximum loudness. My ears are like a microphone that picks up and amplifies sound" (Grandin, 1996b, 1).*

Hypertaste/Hypersmell:

Brad Rand describes his hyperolfactory experience: "Chalk hurts my nose, and soap and perfume and aftershave and toothpaste". He states that for some autistic people "almost all types of food smell too sharp" and they "cannot tolerate" how people smell, even if they are very clean. They do not like some food because "the smell or taste" might be intolerable (Rand, Undated, p. 6). Donna Williams's allergic reaction to some perfumes made the inside of her nose feel like it had been walled up with clay up to her eyebrows, some perfumes "burned her lungs" Williams, 1996, 57). Some autistic individuals have olfactory sensitivities comparable to canines (Morris, 1999, 10).

Hypertactility

is very common among autistic population. For example:

> *"...my fingers felt like they were being torn apart when he (husband) interlocked his fingers with mine... I feel bugs under my skin when he touched me lightly" (Willey, 1999, 66).*
>
> *"Sometimes a nurse would try to hug me or tickle me. This just sent me into a panic attack ...I did not understand why I was afraid of touch but now I think it just caused lots of sensations that were overwhelming for me" (Lawson, 1998, 40-41).*
>
> *"I pulled away when people tried to hug me, because being touched sent an overwhelming tidal wave of stimulation through my body... Small itches and scratches that most people ignore were torture. A scratchy petticoat was like sandpaper rubbing my skin raw. Hair washing was also awful. When my mother scrubbed my hair my scalp hurt" (Grandin, 1996b, 2)*

Gillingham (1991) states that this "superability" of autistic people, when the senses are so finely tuned that they make them acutely aware of things the "normal" person would not notice, sometimes causes extreme pain. Gillingham suggests that to block this pain the body produces endomorphins, that, in turn, may suppress further sensory information.

Hyposensitivity

Hypovision:

"When a sight pathway is not very sensitive, people and objects might be mostly outlines with fuzzy edges. They might have trouble figuring out where objects actually are, so they might walk around something and run their hand around the edges so they can understand exactly where it is... They might even stare at the sun because they don't think it is bright" (Rand, Undated, p.5)

Hypohearing:

"They might lean their ear against the refrigerator to hear the motor vibrating. They might stay in bathrooms a lot because all the sounds echo against the tile and sink and tub. They might like sirens and whistles, squeaky toys, jingling bells, rattling garbage trucks, blasting TVs and stereos, roaring snowblowers, and crashing waves on the beach. They might tear paper or slam doors over and over to hear the sound" (Rand, p. 6)

Hypotaste/Hyposmell:

"I chewed sugar packets whole. I ate school paste and play dough and paraffin... I also enjoyed toilet bowl sanitizing bars and moth balls" (Willey, 1999, 21)

Hypotactility:

"...a piece of that broken glass sliced everything on my forearm all the way to the bone. To the point, I felt nothing, and did not realize that I'd been injured until I glanced down and saw the open, gaping wound and the blood that had gushed all over the front door" (Schneider, 1999, 48)

Delacato (1974) was one of the first to suggest that hyper- and hyposensitivity experienced by autistic children caused all autistic behaviours, viz. withdrawal from social interaction, communication, stereotypic behaviours (or stims, or self-stimulations) which he called sensoryisms (sensorisms: blindisms – visual "isms", deafisms – auditory "isms", etc) and considered them as the child's attempts to treat himself and normalise his sensory channels or communicate his problems.

Autistic individuals often describe their stims as defensive mechanisms from hyper- or hyposensitivity. Sometimes they engage in these behaviours to suppress the pain or calm themselves down (in the case of hypersensitivity), sometimes to arouse the nervous system and get sensory stimulation from the outside (in the case of hyposensitivity), and sometimes to provide themselves with internal pleasure.

The stereotypies caused by sensory hyper- or hyposensitivity can involve one or all senses.

What to look for:

Hyper-	Hypo-
Vision	
1). Constantly looks at minute particles, picks up smallest pieces of dust	1). Is attracted to light
2). Dislikes dark and bright lights	2). Looks intensely at objects or people
3). Notices every tiny change in his environment	3). Moves fingers or objects in front of the eyes
4). Is frightened by sharp flashes of light, lightning, etc.	4). Is fascinated with reflections, bright coloured objects
5). Looks down most of the time	5). Rocking movements
6). Covers or closes eyes at bright light	6). Runs a hand around the edge of the object
7). Makes sudden but controlled movements	7). Perimeter hugging.

Hearing

1). Covers ears

2). Is a very light sleeper

3). Is frightened by animals

4). Dislikes thunderstorm, sea, crowds

5). Dislikes haircut

6). Avoids sounds and noises

7). Makes repetitive noises to block out other sounds

1). Bangs objects, doors

2). Likes vibration

3). Likes kitchen, toilet

4). Likes crowds, traffic, etc.

5). Tears paper, crumples paper in his hand

6). Is attracted by sounds, noises

7). Makes loud rhythmic noises

Taste/Smell

1). Poor eater

2). Uses tip of tongue for tasting

3). Gags/vomits easily

4). Craves certain foods

5). Toiletting problems

6). Runs from smells

7). Wears the same clothes

8). Avoids people

1). Eats anything (pica)

2). Mouths and licks objects

3). Eats mixed food (e.g., sweet and sour)

4). Smells self, people and objects

5). Smears (plays with) faeces

6). Seeks strong odours

7). Bedwetting

8). Regurgitates

Tactility

1). Resists being touched

2). Cannot tolerate new clothes, avoids wearing shoes

3). Overreacts to heat/cold/pain

1). Likes pressure, tight clothes

2). Prone to self-injuries

3). Low reaction to pain and temperature

4). Avoids getting "messy"	4). Places the body in strange positions
5). Dislikes food of certain textures	5). Unaware of his own body sensations
6). Moves away from people	

2. Inconsistency of perception (Fluctuation: between hyper- and hypo-; "falling in/out of")

One of the baffling features of autistic people is their inconsistent perception of sensory stimuli. Here 2 types of this inconsistency are distinguished: fluctuation between hyper- and hypo-; fluctuation between hyper-/hypo- and normal ("in" – "out").

Fluctuation between hyper- and hypo- is widely reported: a child who appears to be deaf on one occasion may react to an everyday sound on another occasion as if it is causing acute pain; visual stimuli that may appear so bright on one occasion will on another occasion appear very dim. Similarly, reaction to pain may vary from complete insensitivity to apparent "over-reaction" to the slightest knock (Jordan & Powell, 1990)

Ornitz and Ritvo (1969) suggest that autism is characterised by fluctuation between states of over and underarousal resulting in a failure to modulate sensory intake adequately and an unstable perceptual experience. The authors argue that the individual's sensitivity to stimuli fluctuates and depends on whether the person Is In a state of over- or underarousal. Ornitz (1989) states that the disturbance of sensory modulation involves all sensory modalities and is manifested as both under- and overreactivity to sensory stimuli and as self-stimulation. The author suggests that optimal levels of stimulation will vary across autistic persons as a function of developmental level, degree of familiarity with the situation, and biologically based individual differences, including the severity of autistic disorder (Ornitz, 1989). This model assumes that the disturbances of sensory modulation are the primary symptoms and the impairments of social interaction, communication, language and bizarre behaviour are consequences of a dysmodulation of sensory input.

In the personal accounts people with autism describe their experience of "unreliable" perception, for example:

> *"Faces began to merge together, voices sounded out of sync and my perception fooled me" (Willey, 1999, 33)*
>
> *"Sometimes when other kids spoke to me I would scarcely hear, then sometimes they sounded like bullets" (White & White, 1987)*
>
> *"It (hearing) gets louder sometimes... Things seem suddenly closer sometimes. Sometimes things get suddenly brighter" (Oliver in Williams, 1994, 189)*
>
> *"It was as though my senses only functioned consistently when I moved within my own world, and that meant closing others out. My mother and father thought I was deaf. Standing behind me, they'd take it in turns to make loud noise without so much as a blink in response... (Hearing test showed) that my hearing was better than average... The problem with my hearing was obviously one of a fluctuation in the awareness of sound. In this case it was as though awareness were a puppet, the string of which were set firmly in the hands of emotional stress" (Williams, 1992, 41)*

Fluctuation between hyper-/hypo- and normal ("in" and "out"). Dr Freeman (1993) describes perception of the world by people with autism "like an FM radio that is not exactly tuned on the station when you are driving down the freeway. Sometimes the world comes in clearly and at other times it does not" (p. 5)

People with autism contribute to the explanation of this phenomenon. Donna Williams compares autism with a seesaw: when it is up or down she cannot see a whole life; when it is passing through in the middle she gets to see a glimpse of the life she would have if she were not autistic (1994, 233). J.G.T.VanDalen terms it as "suddenly falling out of autism" and describes his personal experience of this process as follows: "the stay in the non-autistic condition lasts only a few minutes,.. the exit-procedure occurs instantaneously, the return is gradual" (1995, 13, 14)

Interestingly, it is these experiences that have brought VanDalen to the conclusions that:

- autism is primarily a perceptual deficit as during these short periods when his "perception was normalised" he "noticed above all the diffused fear (he constantly experienced) was completely vanished… the habitual occupation with inanimate physical objects disappeared in favour of all the (warm) feelings that belonged to normal relationships" (p. 13)
- "the degree of autism within an individual can vary considerably even to the point of 'suddenly falling out of it" (p. 13)

What to look for:

Responds differently (indifference – distress) to the same visual/auditory/olfactory/gustatory/tactile stimuli.

3. "Mono-processing"

According to the number of senses working at a time they can be classified into "Multi-Track" versus "Mono"-Processing (Williams, 1996, 95) or "being singly channelled" (Lawson, 1999)

Most people use their senses simultaneously. When they are hearing something, they still continue to make sense of what they see and feel emotionally and physically. They know what their body is doing whilst they are speaking or what their face is doing whilst they are using their hands. They can do all these things because they are "multi-tracked". For people who work in "mono" to process the meaning of what they are listening to whilst being touched may be to have no idea where they were being touched or what they thought or felt about it. To process the location or special significance of being touched whilst someone is showing them something means that they saw nothing but meaningless colour and form and movement (Williams, 1996, 95-96). For example, Donna Williams's inner-body sense, like everything else was mostly in mono: if she touched her leg she would feel it on her hand or on her leg but not both at the same time (Williams, 1994, 228). She had big restrictions in being able to process information from the outside and inside at the same time, for example, touching the furniture she could feel the texture of the wood but would have no sense of her own hand. She could also switch channels and feel her own hand but would lose sensation of what her hand was in contact with. Without being able to process her own body sensations in relations to textures it was, perceptually, as though either "she" did not exist and other things did or they did not exist and "she" did. She was either in a constant state of jolting perceptual shifts or remained on one sensory channel or the other (Williams, 1998, 56).

Jared Blackburn (1999) describes the trouble he had processing many things at once. For example, he could not take notes at the lecture because he could either listen or write, but not both. Many of his teachers thought he was being lazy or inattentive because he did not take notes and did not look at them and had a blank look on his face, but he was actually almost hypnotically focused on what they were saying (p. 8); it is a matter of taking one thing at a time (Kathy French in Donnelly, 1999).

The individuals with autism define this 'mono'-processing as one of their involuntary adaptations to avoid sensory overload. It is a mechanism by which the time and energy that goes into processing gets spread a little less thinly than it otherwise might: switching between different channels gives them an opportunity to keep the remaining ones going more efficiently. It involves no conscious decision or choice, and although one can learn to work with it or against it, it cannot be reasoned with (Williams, 1996; 1998). Donna Williams (1996) illustrates this phenomenon as follows:

> *"This is like having one employee working in a huge department store instead of having a whole staff. If a customer has a demand in the shoe department whilst the worker is presently dealing with a demand in the toy department, the customer in the shoe department wouldn't find anybody there… and sometimes (this single worker closes) the shop in different departments when she can't cope with the demand" (p. 99, 100).*

What to look for:

1) Doesn't seem to see if listening/smelling/feeling taste/touching, etc/

2) Doesn't seem to hear if looking/smelling/feeling taste/touching, etc.

3) Doesn't seem to feel taste if looking/listening/smelling/touching, etc.

4) Doesn't seem to smell if seeing/hearing, etc.

5) Doesn't seem to feel being touched if looking/listening, etc.

6) Fails to define the texture or location of touch.

4. Fragmented perception (perception "in bits", stimulus overselectivity). Partial perception

Very often people with autism are not able to perceive objects, people, and surroundings as a whole. This fragmented perception can affect all the senses:

> *"I had always known that the world was fragmented. My mother was a smell and a texture, my father was a tone, and my older brother was something which was moving about" (Williams, 1992, 11)*

> *"I remember being attracted to pieces of people's faces. I might have liked the color of the eyes, the texture of the hair or the straightness of the teeth" (Willey, 1999, 23)*

> *"Sometimes people would have to repeat a particular sentence several times for me as I would hear it in bits and the way in which my mind had segmented their sentence into words left me with a strange and sometimes unintelligible message. It was a bit like when someone plays around with the volume switch on TV" (Williams, 1992, 61)*

> *"When I was about ten I had begun to hear bits and pieces directly with meaning" (Williams, 1994, 95)*

The perception of parts instead of wholes and utilising only a very limited amount of available information is known as stimulus overselectivity (Lovaas et al., 1971). It results in autistic people often perceiving parts of objects or people as being complete entities:

> *"Where someone else may have seen 'crowd', I saw arm, person, mouth, face, hand, seat, person, eye… I was seeing ten thousand pictures to someone else's one" (Williams, 1998,21)*

> *"I did not see whole. I saw hair, I saw eyes, nose, mouth, chin, …not face" (Alex in Williams, 1999, 180)*

> *"When I am confronted with a hammer, I am initially confronted... with a number of unrelated parts: I notify a cubical piece of iron with its neighborhood a coincidental bar-like piece of wood. After that, I am struck by the coincidental nature of the iron and the wooden thing resulting in the unifying perception of a hammer-like configuration. The name 'hammer' is not immediately within reach but appears when configuration sufficiently stabilized over time. Finally, the use of a tool becomes clear" (VanDalen, 1995, 11)*

One of the theories attempting to explain this phenomenon is the Central coherence theory formulated by Uta Frith (1989) and developed by Francesca Happe (1994). According to this theory people with autism lack the 'built-in form of coherence' (Frith, 1989) and, as a result, they see the world as less integrated, i.e. analytically rather than holistically. One of possible causes for seeing things as disconnected might be lacking the resource(s) to process all relevant parts of a stimulus at once, this, in turn, could result in either overly narrow attentional focus or insufficient memory resources to handle the task (Rand, Undated, 11).

Donna Williams (1996) describes an autistic girl who refuses to look at people, because although she can see an entire person she can only process the meaning of one bit of them at a time and only forms a mental impression from the bits of what she has seen rather than forming coherent mental images. These problems also mean that she finds facial expressions and body language meaningless or even scary, so she generally does not trust people or show much interest in them as people.

This category also includes a sort of 'tunnel vision' experienced by some people with autism:

> *"I pick up his hand and looked at it closely. I traced it with my eyes from the fingers to the shoulder, from the shoulder to the eyes, down to the nose and mouth. Ian was a jigsaw of bits that my mind was in no state to make sense of as a whole" (Williams, 1999, 21)*

This category also includes a permanent condition, viz. *prosopagnosia ("face-blindness")*. Some autistic people are reported to be prosopagnostic (Blackburn, 1999; Grandin, 1996a), i.e. they have trouble recognising people's faces. This condition makes them blind to all but the most familiar faces. The exact effects and severity may vary between people. Temple

Grandin (1996a), for example, often got into embarrassing situations because she did not remember faces unless she had seen the people many times or they had a very distinct facial feature, such as a big beard, thick glasses or a strange hairstyle (p. 74).

Some experimental studies of autistic people's capacity to process faces suggest that they use abnormal processing strategies and experience less difficulties when faces are presented to them upside-down. Whether it is true for their perception of the whole environment needs further investigation.

Non-autistic prosopagnostics state that face blindness tends to isolate them from people in general, as being unable to recognise others interferes with making and maintaining relationships (Bill, 1997). They work out their own recognition system. Most common features that seem to work best for face blind people are: casual clothes, long hair and facial hair, and movement. Bill (1997), who is face blind, describes his method to recognise people by their jeans, movements and hair (as the inability to recognise faces does not extend to hair, particularly if it is long enough to extend out of the face area). He can see a pattern in hair texture and process hairlines. Interestingly, that many autistic people are reported to be fascinated by people's hair, and many do not recognise their relatives if they wear unfamiliar clothes.

As some individuals with autism perceive everything in pieces they need time to adjust to different surroundings. As the number of objects seen by them is greater because they see different images of one and the same object from different angles (VanDalen, 1995), they do not feel safe in this chaos of things and people. As a consequence of this fragmented perception autistic individuals exhibit maintenance of sameness, resistance to change, anxiety in unfamiliar places.

The mechanism of unrelated "points-of-view" is illustrated by VanDalen (1995):

> *"when I approach a familiar street by accident from an unusual direction, I do not immediately recognise my homely environment" (p.12)*

Sensing in bits results in autistic individuals defining people and places and things by these bits and therefore they can suddenly find once familiar things to be strikingly unfamiliar if slight components are changed, such as when someone moves the furniture or does not wear the same coat as usual (Williams, 1996). For instance, when Donna Williams was a child and because she processed what she saw piece by piece and not as a whole, she knew her mother by her tone, pace and smell. If someone else smelled like her, had sharp movements and spoke with a similar tone, Donna responded to them as though they were her mother. At the big supermarkets she kept latching on to strangers because they wore the same colour or fabrics as her mother on that day. She was always horrified when 'her mother' did not make sense because the wrong type of hair would be attached to the clothes or she would be moving in a way that was not hers. She had gone to the wrong houses because they had an important identifying component but gradually everything else did not fit (Williams, 1996, 182-183).

Another 'side-effect' of perception in bits is "a sense of fear that is not specifically related to certain objects but is originated in the fact that (the) first encounter with a physical object is a partial one" (VanDalen, 1995,12).VanDalen compares this experience with a confrontation with a silhouette in the dark: one knows that something is there but it is not altogether immediately clear what it is.

What to look for:

1). Resists any change

2). Gets frustrated if there is a tiny change in the environment

3). Selects for attention minor aspects of objects in the environment instead of the whole scene

4). Gets lost easily

5). Does not recognise people in unfamiliar clothes, on photographs

6). Hears a few words instead of the whole sentence

7). Complains about some parts of the clothes, smells of some pieces of food, etc.

5. Distorted perception

Although fragmented perception can be also termed distorted, here distorted perception means not fragmentation but rather change (distortion) in the perception of the form, space sound, etc. For example, hearing distorted sounds or hearing intonation rather than words:

> *"I hear SOUNDS rather than WORDS... Sometimes I ...forget a message, but remember the tonal quality" (Blackburn, 1999)*

> *"I'd get the intonation but lose the meaning of the words or get the meaning of the words but only at the cost of tuning out the intonation, as though independent of the words" (Williams, 1998, 63)*

In the field of vision the most common distortions reported by the individuals with autism are: poor/distorted depth and space perception, seeing 2D world, 'double vision', distortions of shape, size, movement, etc. For example:

> *"I used to hate small shops because my eyesight used to make them look as if they were even smaller than they actually are" (White & White, 1987, 223)*

Van Dalen (1995) says that his space seems to be expanded and a single room bears the same spatial characteristics as a whole house.

Autistic individuals often have problems with understanding boundaries and relationships between objects in space and their own body; sometimes they are confused about the parts of their bodies. For example, Oliver (in Williams, 1994, 191) describes his experiences of "losing his legs": "I had no sense of my body from my waist down. I feel like I was flying". As a teenager, Donna Williams spent many hours trying to shake a hand off an arm without the perception that both were part of her body (1996, 14).

Sometimes they experience difficulties in perception of movement:

> *"...the crowd's constant commotion and moving about made me feel light-headed and disoriented" (Willey, 1999, 66)*

> *"Occasionally I lost all sense of perspective. Something would seem monstrously large if coming towards me at speed, or if I was unprepared.*

Someone suddenly leaning over me could frighten me enormously. I felt something was falling onto me and that I'd be crushed underneath it " (Gerland, 1997)

"The bitumen floor of the school playground intrigued me and I noticed that as I ran it seemed to run with me" (Lawson, 1998, 29)

One of characteristic behaviours of autistic children is to spin themselves and enjoy swings without becoming dizzy. The individuals with autism report that these activities help them normalise perception and a vestibular system. For example, for Donna Williams, compulsive and repetitive spinning, jumping from heights, climbing to great heights and throwing herself backwards onto things and falling through space were attempts to develop a vestibular system that was not able to work consistently or efficiently (1996, 127).

Russell (1994) suggested that one of basic deficits in autism might be disturbance at the stage of "efferent copying": In normal development the 'efferent copying' gives the sense of one's own agency, i.e., the nervous system does not only control movements of the head and eyes to scan the environment or keep track of moving objects, but also records those movements in order to distinguish the case where the movement is in the person's head and eyes, and the world is still. In autism, the researcher suggests, the disturbance at the stage of 'efferent copying' prevents the person from having a sense of themselves as an agent. In this case the person would not get dizzy in the normal way from spinning and, moreover, he might seek for the kinds of sensations that would give movement stimulation free from recording head and eye movements in relation to the world.

Distortions are reported to become worse in the state of nervous overarousal and information overload.

What to look for:

1). Compulsive repetitive hand, head or body movements that fluctuate between near and far

2). Fears heights, stairs, escalators

3). Has difficulty catching balls

4). Appears startled when being approached

5). Climbs high into a tree, jumps off tall fences, etc.

6). Gets lost easily

7). Enjoys swings, merry-go-rounds

8). Spins, runs round and round

9). Hits eyes/ears/nose/oneself

10). Unable to distinguish between some sounds

6. Peripheral perception. Avoidance of central/direct perception.

One of the characteristics of autism is avoidance of eye contact. Here it is included in the category of peripheral perception, as it turns out that avoidance of direct perception is not restricted only to vision but also includes other sensory systems.

One of the theories (Delacato, 1974) to account for this feature is that people with autism use peripheral vision because their central vision is hypo while their peripheral vision is hyper. However analysis of the personal accounts of individuals with autism shows that often they do not use their direct/central perception because "it hurts", i.e. it is hyper. For instance, for Nony eye contact was painful: "It was not quite like a broken bone or a burn but it can only be described as pain" (1993).

Jean-Paul Bovee describes eye contact as something that he always had trouble with, as all of the stress that is put on doing it makes him more nervous, tense, and scared (Bovee, Undated, p.2).

Jasmine O'Neill reports that "gazing directly at people or animals is many times too overwhelming... Some autistic people don't even look at the eyes of actors or news reporters on television" (O'Neill, 1999, 26).

Some of the problems autistics have with making eye contact may be nothing more than an intolerance for the movement of the other person's eyes. Temple Grandin writes about one autistic person for whom looking at other people's eyes was difficult because the eyes did not stay still (1996a, 73).

Donna Williams states that connections, which are too direct, hurt (1994, 44), because often direct perception is hyper and it brings sensory overload resulting in a switching to 'mono':

> "*I actually hear you better when I am not looking at you... eye contact is... uncomfortable... (people) will never understand the battle I have gone through to be able to do this. I can understand why Aboriginal people believe eye contact destroys the soul of their ancestors" (Lawson, 1998, 11, 12)*

Donna Williams explains that when taking things indirectly, peripherally, the fragmentation did not happen; things were more cohesive, they retained context, whereas the mind-jolting senses of direct vision and direct hearing could not be consistently relied upon as meaningful primary senses (1998, 63).

Some autistic people seem to be hypersensitive when they are approached directly by other people:

> "*Dr Marek was 'touching' me with his eyes... I was afraid... I was being hurt" (Williams, 1994, 121)*

> "*It can feel creepy to be searched with the eyes" (O'Neill, 1999, 26)*

> "*Someone looking directly into my eyes felt like an attack" (Nony, 1993)*

Avoidance of direct perception for them is another involuntary adaptation that helps them to survive in a sensory distorted world:

> "*A form of instinctual closing out of visual information is the involuntary turning in of one eye or staring through things which has the effect of putting visual information temporarily out of focus and, therefore, decreases visual information overload" (Williams, 1996, 126).*

Donna Williams (1996, 41) describes an autistic girl who can often make better meaning out of what she hears or sees by looking or listening peripherally (such as out of the corner of her eye or by looking at or listening to something else). In this case it is a kind of indirectly-confrontational approach in contrast to 'normal' directly-confrontational one (Williams, 1998). Indirectly-confrontational communication can mean that if something needs explaining or showing, the person explaining or showing can do so as if out loud to themselves, addressing the wall or the floor, or one's shoes, or the objects relating to the demonstration. The person with a problem of overload should be allowed, similarly, to address and interact with you through speaking out loud with you 'in mind'. Gradually, bridges can be built from indirectly to more directly confrontational interaction and communication (Williams, 1996, 118)

The same is true for other senses if they are hypersensitive: indirect perception of smell or 'instrumental touch' (Williams, 1994) are often defensive mechanisms to avoid overload.

When hypersensitivity of the affected sensory channel is addressed and lessened, the direct perception becomes easier. For example, by wearing Irlen tinted glasses that helped eliminate her visual hypersensitivity Donna Williams realised that now she absorbed far more direct visual information:

> *"Everything that was taken peripherally before was now being taken in directly. But overload didn't happen; everything seemed more contained, more controlled, less invasive and frightening" (Williams, 1999, 176).*

What to look for:

1). Avoids direct eye contact

2). Reacts to the instructions when they are 'addressed to the wall'

3). Can tolerate only 'instrumental' (not 'social') touch

4). Avoids direct smell/taste

7. Inability to distinguish between foreground and background stimuli (Inability to filter foreground and background)

Delacato (1974) discovered that autistic children ("hypervisual" in his classification) are not fooled by optical illusions and identified it as one of the visual "isms". There have appeared several theories attempting to account for this phenomenon: the theory of "prediction of probabilities" (Feigenberg, 1986) and the modification of the "weak coherence theory" (Frith, 1989) to low levels (Happe,1996).

Some people with autism experience an inability to filter out irrelevant visual information and cannot distinguish between foreground and background stimuli. This may account for their 'superability' to see simultaneously two pictures in one (e.g., 'vase-faces' picture). Other 'disillusions' (e.g., Titcher circles, etc.) can be accounted for by 'prediction of probabilities' deficit (Feigenberg, 1986).

This phenomenon, termed here as "optical disillusion", is included into a broader category, covering all the senses, viz. inability to distinguish between foreground and background visual/auditory/olfactory/gustatory/ tactile stimuli. The analysis of the personal accounts shows that this inability to filter foreground and background sensory stimuli is quite common among autistic population. For example:

Vision: "...what was background to others had been foreground to me...everything was taken in peripherally without judgement, filtration or selection" (Williams, 1999, 198)

"The relatedness of things disappeared and everything was now conceptually a separate and unrelated entity. The 'on' and 'next' and 'in front of' didn't mean much anymore, because whatever something was 'on', 'next to' or 'in front of' no longer had a reality until it itself was focused upon directly" (Williams, 1999, 211-212)

Hearing: Temple Grandin is unable to talk on the telephone in a noisy office or airport. If she tries to screen out the background noise, she also screens out the voice on the telephone (1996b).

When two people are talking at once, it is difficult for her to screen out one voice and listen to the other, her ears pick up all sound with equal intensity (1996a, 68)

Touch: "It is hard to have someone touch you when you can't make proper consistent sense of where all your parts are or where you and the room and other people begin and end" (Williams, 1999, 33)

What to look for:

1). Is not fooled by optical illusions

2). Gets frustrated when trying to do something in a noisy or crowded room

3). Unable to distinguish between strong and weak tactile/gustatory/olfactory stimuli

8. Sensitivity to (disturbance by) certain sensory stimuli

This category differs from hypersensitivity in that it is narrower and includes disturbance only by certain stimuli while being indifferent or fascinated by others, although in any case the senses should be hypersensitive to experience it. The kind of stimuli that are disturbing vary from person to person. A sight, sound, etc that cause one child pain may be pleasurable to another.

Jasmine L.O'Neill (1999) compares the sensitivity of autistics to certain stimuli with allergies:

> *"It's at the point of being overwhelmed that it can feel as if you're allergic... (autistic reactions to some stimuli) can seem like allergies on the surface" (pp. 93, 94)*

All senses can be affected. For example, Liane H.Willey (1999) found many noises and bright lights nearly impossible to bear:

> *"Whistles, party noisemakers, flutes and trumpets and any close relative of these sounds disarmed my calm and made my world very uninviting.*

> *Bright lights, mid-day sun, reflected lights, strobe lights, flickering lights; each seemed to sear my eyes" (p. 22)*

Wendy Lawson (1998) reports that certain noises and the pitch of some sounds cause her a lot of discomfort:

> *"The buzzer on the microwave oven, children's voices, car horns, the bus bell people activate to tell the driver they want to get off, a kettle whistling… these are just some of the sounds I find unbearable" (p. 4)*

Many autistic individuals emphasise that not only certain sound but any sudden unpredictable sounds can be painful:

> *"Sudden loud noises hurt my ears – like a dentist's drill hitting a nerve" (Grandin, 1992)*
>
> *"I jumped out of my skin when animals made noises" (White & White, 1987)*

The fear of noise that hurts the ears is often the cause of many bad behaviours and tantrums. Some autistic children, for instance, could break the telephone because they are afraid it will ring (Grandin, 1996b). Some autistic people often find it impossible to touch some objects:

> *"I hated stiff things, satiny things, scratchy things…" (Willey, 1999, 21)*

Donna Williams calls one of her particular texture problems 'wool on wool', i.e. intolerance when hair rubbing against hair or cloth against cloth. It means that it is difficult to her to tolerate people's hair rubbing on her or their clothes rubbing her clothes, and it is hard to tolerate putting woollen jumper over her head or walking on some carpets with certain types of socks, etc. (Williams, 1996).

The most often reported visual sensitivities are: sensitivity to bright light, fluorescent light, colours and certain patterns (especially, stripes).

The light sensitivity in autism coincides completely with the symptoms of Scotopic Sensitivity/Irlen Syndrome (SS/IS) identified by Helen Irlen (1991).

Many autistic people confirm that bright lights and sunshine disturb them and often cause distortions. For example, as a child, Nony (1993) found it difficult to walk in town on a sunny day; her eyes would close and she would have to turn into a darker doorway or cover her eyes to get them open enough to see; the glare of sidewalks and shop windows was too much for her. Some people report that on bright days the sight blurs (White & White, 1987).

Fluorescent light has been reported by many autistic individuals to be very difficult to tolerate, because they can see a sixty-cycle flicker. Problems with flickering can range from excessive eyestrain to seeing a room pulsate on and off (Grandin, 1996a, 75). For example, Donna Williams was tortured by sharp white fluorescent light which made reflections bounce off everything: it made the room busily in a constant state of change, light and shadows dancing on people's faces as they spoke turned the scene into an animated cartoon (Williams, 1994, 74). Sara Miller (in Donnelly, 1999) says that when fluorescent lights are flickering, it takes her attention away from what she is trying to do.

Reported strategies to cope with light sensitivity are: turning off any unnecessary lighting (especially, fluorescent lightning), mat surfaces on walls, lamps rather than overhead lights, low wattage light bulbs, Irlen lenses, etc.

Sensitivity to colours and colour contrast is another visual problem for some autistic people. For example:

> *"I find pastels difficult to look at... my mouth fills with saliva and my head hurts. They make me feel icky, queasy, uneven. I can take them in small doses, in crayon boxes or mixed in a fabric that is based in a darker color, but I do not like to feel immersed in them. They drown me" (Willey, 1999, 92)*

> *"The kitchen had fluorescent lights and yellow walls, one of the worst combinations ever. Even from the doorway I could see light bouncing off everything" (Williams, 1994, 92)*

What to look for:

1). Squints or closes eyes in bright light.

2). Gets easily frustrated/tired under fluorescent lights

3). Gets frustrated with certain colours

4). Gets frustrated with certain sounds

5). Tries to destroy/break objects producing sounds (clock, telephone, toy, etc.)

6). Cannot tolerate certain textures

7). Cannot tolerate some smells/tastes

9. Fascination with certain stimuli

This is an opposite of disturbance by certain stimuli, caused also by hypersensitivity. These two features are like two sides of one and the same coin. The only difference is while disturbance causes pain, fascination gives pleasant experiences and brings calm and peace to autistic people, although at the cost of their withdrawal.

Sometimes people with autism, when they have given up fighting in an incomprehensible world, rescue themselves from overload to an entertaining, secure and hypnotic level of hyper: watching the reflection of every element of light and colour, tracing every patterned shape and vibration of noise as it bounces off the walls (Williams, 1994, 112). Donna Williams names it as the beautiful side of autism, sanctuary of the prison. She describes how she would wander through the school, watching the various colours which disappeared under her feet and she would stop sometimes and stare at something like the polished floor or the reflection in the curved tinted-glass window.

Jasmine O'Neill says that autistic people can be fascinated with different sensory stimuli, such as the smell of melting candles, rice cooking, the feel of velvet and marble, the taste of smooth, satiny wood, the pit-pat of bare feet on tiles, the look of clouds gliding high, the feel of a horse's nose, the chalky taste of seashells (1999, 28).

The sources of fascinations are very individual. For example, to Liane H.Willey (1999) such visual elements as linear lines, symmetry, balance, straightness, perfect alignments, squares and triangles were appealing. Wendy Lawson (1998) finds certain colours fascinating. Her favourite colours are rich emerald green, royal blue, purple, turquoise. A typical picture of an individual with autism is when he is sitting staring transfixed at the crystal, turning it around and around in front of his eyes, catching rainbows (Oliver in: Williams, 1994, 189).

What to look for:

1). Is fascinated with coloured and shining objects

2). Is fascinated with certain sounds

3). Is fascinated with certain tastes/smells

4). Is fascinated with certain textures

10. "Losing oneself" in certain stimuli. "Resonance"

These terms were introduced by Donna Williams (1994; 1996; 1998; 1999) to define a state when one 'loses oneself' in/becoming resonant with something else. Here they are used to denote the higher degrees of fascination with sensory stimuli. The person can merge with (lose oneself in) different sensory stimuli. For example, a petal of a rose triggers the feeling of merging with the smell of it:

> *"My nose zoomed in on (bits of the petal) like a camera taking a photograph and I took a long breath. I was swept up in the smell, becoming part of the rose it had come from" (Williams, 1994, 4)*

Wendy Lawson describes her experience when the colours and fragrance were so vibrant to her senses that she could 'feel' them. While watching some shiny things she felt a sense of connection, she felt safe, as if she were part of them: "It was so intoxicating and I felt so alive" (1998, 2).

Donna Williams describes how she could 'feel' colours:

> *"These streetlights were yellow with a hint of pink but in a buzz state they were an intoxicating iridescent-like pink-yellow. My mind dived deeper and deeper into the colour, trying to feel its nature and become it as I progressively lost sense of self in its overwhelming presence. Each of the colours resonated different feelings within me and it was like they played me as a chord, where other colours played one note at a time.*

> *It had been the same as long as I had known... some things hadn't changed... since I was an infant swept up in the perception of swirling air particles, a child lost in the repetition of a pattern of sound, or a teenager staring for hours at coloured billiard balls, trying to grasp the experience of the particular colour I was climbing into" (1999, 19)*

Willey loved the sensation that came from floating with water: she felt as if she was liquid, tranquil, smooth (1999, 22).

In the state of 'resonance' one can sense the surface, texture and density of material without looking at it with physical eyes or touching it with physical hands or tasting it without a physical tongue or tapping it to hear it sounds, i.e. sensing it with non-physical senses (the so-called 'shadow senses') (Williams, 1999, 36-37).

Those who experience this condition can be 'in resonance' with colours, sounds, objects, places, plants, animals, people, etc. E.g.:

> *"I could resonate with the cat and spent hours lying in front of it, making no physical contact with it. I could resonate with the tree in the park and feel myself merge with its size, its stability, its calm and its flow" (Williams, 1998, 44)*

'In resonance' with people they can sense ('see', 'hear' etc.) thoughts, emotions, pain, etc of other people, e.g.:

> *"It is rare that I know what anyone is actually thinking, but concurrent emotions are very common" (McKean, 1994)*
>
> *"When I was younger I heard a lot of noises in my head, spoken things and unspoken things. Tell me you can hear people think. I wish I didn't. If there is a medication that will kill people's thoughts I like to try it" (Walker & Cantello, 1994)*
>
> *"I physically felt the pain when someone banged themselves. Around someone with a broken leg, I felt their pain in my leg" (Williams, 1998, 59)*
>
> *"I ...remember responding to people's call by coming into the room, sometimes answering their request by going and getting what they'd wanted. People had seemed surprised at these behaviours because they*

> *hadn't been verbally called or asked or that I was busy with things of my own at the time" (Williams, 1998, 27)*

Similar experiences have been reported by few other autistic individuals. Probably, some people are reluctant to share these experiences because there is always a fear of being considered 'psychic'.

Interestingly, cats and dogs seem to possess a similar sort of 'telepathic' ability. Sheldrake (1999) suggests it could be caused by some force field ('morphic field') that is not yet fully understood.

Donna Williams (1998) offers her explanation of the phenomenon: The body is more than a physical form. It is also an energy form. Some people's energy boundaries are more 'open' than for most people. These are the people most prone to a wider range of 'psychic' experiences and 'déjà vu'. This state is involuntary, beyond their control. They can either give in to it or try to fight it.

What to look for:

These experiences are very difficult to be identified by 'outsiders'. There are two main reasons for this:

i) even high-functional verbal autistic children often see no need to describe these experiences as they assume that others experience the same

ii) autistic adults are often very unwilling to talk about these in order not to sound crazy or psychic.

However, it may be that many parents do feel that their children are able to 'read their minds' (not to be confused with the 'theory of mind'), but they are also afraid to articulate their suspicions. Indeed, I have met two mothers who confided in me about their feelings. Other indicators can be:

1) Seems to be absorbed with lights, colours, sounds, smells, etc.

2) Seems to feel pain of others.

11. Daydreaming.

It is not uncommon among autistic people to experience the so-called 'daydreams'. Whether this phenomenon is the sixth sense, clairvoyance, precognition or other form of extra-sensory perception and whether we can explain it or not, it does exist. Personal accounts of autistic individuals contain quite a number of these experiences, e.g.:

> *"At school strange things were happening. I would have daydreams in which I was watching children I knew. I would see them doing the trivialest of things: peeling potatoes over the sink, getting themselves a peanut butter sandwich before going to bed. Such daydreams were like films in which I'd see a sequence of everyday events which really didn't relate in any way to myself. I began to test the truth of these daydreams; approaching the friends I'd seen in them and asking them to give me a step-by-step detailed picture of what they were doing at the time I had the daydream. Amazingly, to the finest detail, I had been right. This was nothing I had controlled, it simply came into my head, but it frightened me" (Williams, 1992, 63)*

> *"There were odd occasions at school when I seemed to know things about people before they did. One day when two children were skipping rope and the game was getting intense, I knew that one child would fall down – I had hardly seen the thought when it happened. I know this could easily be coincidence, but it happened many times. Sometimes I would dream of a place, in great detail, and then experience that very same place at some future time" (Lawson, 1998, 30)*

Donna Williams emphasises that these are not fantasies, these are real experiences, which she calls "unintentional out-of-body experiences" (1998):

> *"In my teens I lived in quite a dangerous and lonely state a lot of the time and this caused me to 'visit' non-physically people and places where I felt safe. I didn't fantasize what I'd like to say or do. I simply found myself feeling physically in these places or with these people… Yet I did feel myself moving up the stairs to my friend's flat, through the front door and into the kitchen. I could sense the smell of the room and the noises in the room. I could 'hear' and 'see' as my friends moved about and went on with things" (p. 34)*

What to look for:

There are no general indications to this phenomenon. However, bearing in mind that it is possible, one might find that some behaviours or attempts to explain something 'just fit'.

12 Delayed perception (delayed processing).

It is not uncommon for autistic children to exhibit delayed responses to stimuli:

> *"As a child,.. it appeared as though I didn't feel pain or discomfort, didn't want help, didn't know what I was saying, didn't listen or didn't watch. By the time some of these sensations, responses or comprehensions were decoded and processed for meaning and personal significance, and I'd accessed the means of responding, I was fifteen minutes, one day, a week, a month, even a year away from the context in which the experiences happened" (Williams, 1996, 90)*

Concerning vision, VanDalen (1995) attempts to give one of the possible explanations of this phenomenon: the acquisition of the full meaning requires some observation time from different points of view; besides, people with autism must translate perceptual configurations into their proper terminology. Thus, autistic people "experience meaning on the end of the long road of perception". VanDalen uses the term "photometaphor" which means that autistic people are suffering from a prolonged exposure time producing many blurred pictures. To minimise this detrimental effect, the scene to be photographed must be frozen for some time; for them static pictures are often more impressive than the dynamic reality.

The experience of 'delayed hearing' is termed by B.Rimland as 'delayed mental audition' (1964): when the question has been sensed and recorded without interpretation until the second (internalised) hearing. Thus, Jared Blackburn (1999, 33) often needs some time to process the question and his response. (Immediate responses are often given on 'autopilot', triggered by 'serial memories' – see 19). Before proper response autistic people must go through a number of separate stages in perception, and if this long decision-chain is interrupted by the outside world, the autistic person must start all over again because overselectivity has changed the scene completely (VanDalen, 1995).

Rimland describes the effect of 'delayed mental audition' as an echo; and the sound of the echo-like voice is high-pitched, hollow and parrot-like, i.e. the internally experienced voice duplicates precisely the classical manner of speech of an autistic child. Rimland names it the 'closed loop' phenomenon when the stimuli enter memory and later emerge unchanged (1964, 178-179).

A person can be delayed on every sensory channel. The result is that it takes time to make meaning of or to label, or find personal significance to do with what the person experiences (Williams, 1996, 142).

There are several consequences. One of them is, that new experiences, no matter how similar to previous ones, are perceived as new, unfamiliar and unpredictable, and responses to them are poor regardless of the number of times the person has experienced the same thing. Another one is that as the amount of time needed to process any experience often remains slow (or delayed) regardless of having had similar experiences in the past, things do not get easier with time or learning (Williams, 1996, 143). For example, every situation that Wendy Lawson encounters is like encountering it for the first time. She tends to not take what she has learnt from one situation and be able to apply it to another (1999, 4).

What to look for:

1). Response to visual/auditory/gustatory/olfactory/tactile stimuli is delayed

2). Echolalia in monotonous, high-pitched, parrot-like voice

3). Any experiences are perceived as new and unfamiliar, regardless of the number of times the person has experienced the same thing.

13. Vulnerability to sensory overload

Many autistic people are very vulnerable to sensory overload. They may become overloaded in situations that would not bother other people

(Blackburn, 1997; Lawson, 1998; Morris, 1999; Lawson, 1998; Willey, 1999). The causes of information of overload can be:

- the inability to filter out irrelevant, or excessive information,
- delayed processing,
- if the person works in 'mono' but is forced to attend to the information from several channels,
- distorted perception, resulting in anxiety, confusion, frustration and stress, that, in turn, leads to hypersensitivity.

Donna Williams emphasises that sensory hypersensitivity can happen both independently of information overload and as a direct result of it (1996, 200). The overload can result in hypersensitivity (with its resulting physical pain, tantrums and difficult behaviour). Sometimes it can go to 'accumulation of unknown knowing', i.e. when information gets processed outside of conscious awareness so that one is not aware of what one knows nor able consciously or voluntarily to access that knowledge, though, sometimes it can be triggered or cued by something outside (Williams, 1996, 100); or might go further to 'total systems shutdowns' (Williams, 1996; Blackburn, 1997) (See Descriptor 14).

The process from hypersensitivity to systems shutdowns may be fast, i.e. sensory discomfort may be short lasting or not experienced at all, or may be slow, i.e. sensory discomfort may be prolonged.

The information overload may be diffused before it leads to systems shutdowns or it may not. In the first case, a person may experience severe sensory heightening, colours becoming too intense, light becoming too bright, certain pitches becoming intolerable, certain patterns becoming obtrusively distinct, touch may feel 'prickly' or 'ticklish', or provoke 'shock', yet continue to process information. If information overload is not diffused in time, there may be a temporary inability to process touch, sound or visual information (Williams, 1996, 217). For example:

> *"Overload had set in. Explanations were just blah- blah- blah… My vision started to climb… The lights became brighter. I was tickled by the effect on my senses and began to giggle. The hypersensitivity… climbed even higher… I squinted and grinned, the strain and the confusion of the sudden change from happy to excited to tortured took place within*

> *the space of fifteen minutes with no cues to tell me why or what I was feeling and no time to reflect. My ship was sinking and no one knew" (Williams, 1994, 106).*

> *"Together, the sharp sounds and the bright lights were more than enough to overload my senses. My head would feel tight, my stomach would churn, and my pulse would run my heart ragged until I found a safety zone" (Willey, 1999, 22).*

The causes of information overload on auditory level are reported not to do with the perception of pitch and volume but rather with the number of simultaneous sound sources, the duration of these stimuli and the rate of the bombardment relative to process capacity. Then hearing becomes acute, sounds that are normally inaudible can be as audible as usual sounds, the perception of these additional sounds can make them intensely unbearable (Williams, 1996, 60, 202). Donna Williams considers this reverberation of sound as one of the biggest contributors to sound information overload.

The visual equivalent of sound reverberation, according to Donna Williams, is light refraction (or 'shine') that can cause a visual effect of shooting out streams or 'sparks' of light and 'visually cutting up' people and objects (1996, 112). The same can happen with touch: when too much of visual and auditory information has been taken in, the sense of touch can be oversensitive, "sharp as a pin", and to be touched can be "shocking" (Williams, 1996, 202).

Donna Williams compares a person with a problem of overload with one worker who is being shouted at without warning from too many directions all at once; the worker is bound to be unable to meet all the demands sufficiently and will not have time to work out priorities; when the worker gets overloaded too much, she throws the job in. If only those jobs that need her to attend to them are presented one at a time, the worker will be able to cope for longer (Williams, 1996, 109).

The threshold for processing sensory stimuli varies among autistic persons, at different ages and in different environments. For example:

> *"When I was a small child, my threshold for processing blah-blah was only a few seconds. When I was about ten or so, my threshold… was about five to ten minutes. When I was a teenager and up to my*

> *twenties, this threshold was about fifteen minutes to half an hour. Now it is about twenty to forty-five minutes. In a more accommodating environment… these thresholds could have been much higher than they were" (Williams, 1996, 204).*

Dena Gitlitz (in Donnelly, 1999) names it Eight Ball Theory: Eight Ball is similar to a juggler that can successfully juggle 7 pins or balls but if you throw in one more they will drop them all. Dena has a limited capacity for "how many balls she can juggle" successfully.

This phenomenon could be called the "rule of the last drop": if the child's inner 'cup' is full already, whatever the reasons for this may be, a slightest trigger, which on the days when the 'cup' is empty would not be noticed by the child, might produce an overload.

Each individual may cope with overstimulating stimuli in different ways: 'mono' processing, avoidance of direct perception, withdrawal, stereotypies, etc.

What to look for:

1). Sudden outbursts of self-abuse/tantrums/difficult behaviours.

2). Withdrawal.

14. Systems shutdowns

Too much sensory overload may result in systems shutdowns, in which the person loses some or all of the normal functioning. Shutdown may feel different to different people, but is extremely unpleasant (Blackburn, 1997, 2).

Systems shutdowns may be considered as an involuntary adaptation (compensation) when the brain put certain systems of functioning off limits to improve the level of functioning in others (Williams, 1996, 129). Donna Williams distinguishes three basic forms of system shutdowns:

1. *Shutdown in the ability to simultaneously process sensory information and thought, feeling, body sensation or the monitoring intentional and voluntary expression:* All processing capacity may be diverted to processing incoming sensory information and no connections may be made to

responding to that information. Donna Williams calls this state "all other, no self". For example, Temple Grandin (1996a, 44) remembers how at the age of three she was frustrated because although she could understand what people said to her, she could not get her words out. On the other hand, incoming information, which has previously been processed, may be responded to at the expense of not being able to further process any more information ("all self, no other").

2. *Shutdown in the ability to simultaneously process sensory information on several channels at once:* Donna Williams subdivides it into temporary partial and extended systems shutdowns. Temporary systems shutdowns works by shutting down the ability to process information on a number of channels so that information can be efficiently processed on whatever channel or channels are remaining. Temporary systems shutdowns can affect the processing and monitoring of body awareness, touch, taste, smell, vision or hearing. They can be partial or almost total for any one sense. Partial shutdown means that only a percentage of processing may fall out of a particular sense (partial meaning deafness, partial meaning blindness, partial touch deadness, etc.), for example, a high-functioning person with autism (Jim) could work with overload and shutdown in a way that never left him with any one system shut down permanently but left the forfeiting of systems in a constant state of shift (Jim in: Williams, 1994, 183). Total shutdowns mean that though, for instance, eyes continue to see and ears to hear, the brain does not process any meaning of what is being seen or heard. Temple Grandin (1996a) calls these states as visual tuneouts or whiteouts and auditory tuneouts. Extended systems shutdowns are where a particular systems shutdown is a compensation to handle information overload over an extended amount of time: days, weeks and, very occasionally, a few months and even years.
3. *Temporary or extended shutdown in the ability to maintain conscious and voluntary processing* leads to the accumulation of the 'unknown knowing' (See Descriptor 13).

What to look for:

1). Appears to be a mindless follower

2). Surprises with knowing 'unknown' information

3). Limited ability to gather information on a particular channel

4). Anxiety and depression, insecurity and lack of confidence.

15. "Sensory agnosia" (Blackburn, 1997) (difficulty interpreting a sense).

Donna Williams (1994; 1996; 1998; 1999) calls this experience "meaning-blind/meaning-deaf/touch-dead". She compares this condition with being deaf-blind; the main difference being: the blind get meaning without seeing, while the meaning-blind see without meaning. The deaf-blind may have lost their sense but the meaning-blind/deaf lost the sense (meaning) (Williams, 1994; 1998).

'Blind while seeing' (VanDalen, 1995), 'deaf while hearing', etc. can happen either after overload or after 'losing oneself' in some stimuli, for example:

> *(after overload): "I looked at the beige-colored rectangular blob in front of me. Meaning had shut down not only through my ears but now through my eyes, too. I could see it but I had absolutely no idea what it was for anymore" (Williams, 1994, 106-107).*
>
> *('lost in' a haunting, blue square): "I had fallen into meaning-blindness, and my visual hypersensitivity was absolutely sky-high without any interpretation at all but I had been too hypnotized by beauty to notice it coming up" (Williams, 1994, 222).*

In the state of sensory agnosia interpretation of any sense can be lost; they often act as if they were really blind, deaf, numb, sometimes 'dead'. It is a very frightening experience. Each individual develops his/her own strategies to cope with it.

What to look for:

1). Feels/acts blind/deaf/etc.

2). Displays ritualistic behaviours.

16. Compensating for unreliable senses by other senses.

Because of hypersensitivity, fragmented, distorted perception, delayed processing, sensory agnosia, inability to filter irrelevant stimuli, one sense is never enough for autistic people to make sense of their environment. Thus, in the case of visual distortions and meaning-blindness, they use their ears, nose, tongue or hand to 'see', i.e. they compensate their temporary 'blindness' through other senses. For example, Donna Williams used to tap objects to produce the sound and test their nature, because visual recognition often remained a fragmented and meaningless system. She knew rooms by sound and movement, i.e. she made special repetitive or sudden testing noises in certain rooms and this confirmed the familiarity of a room or its similarity to other rooms. Another means of testing the familiarity of objects, places and people for her was smell and the way an object gave way when bitten (1998, 62):

> *"Ian was a jigsaw of bits that my mind was in no state to make sense of as a whole. I put his hand to my face and smell it: familiarity…I touched the wispy strands (of his hair) and smelled: familiarity. 'Ian's hair', I exclaimed" (Williams, 1999, 21)*

To many autistic people the senses of touch and smell are more reliable (Joan & Rich, 1999, 3).

Many autistic children touch and smell things, some constantly tap everything to figure out where the boundaries are in their environment, like a blind person tapping with a cane. Their eyes and ears function, but they are not able to process incoming visual and auditory information (Grandin, 1996a).

Therese Joliffe preferred using touch to learn about her environment and get a relatively accurate representation of the world, because her vision and hearing were distorted and gave her unreliable information; she 'saw' the world mostly through her fingers (Joliffe et al., 1992).

What to look for:

Tests visual/auditory/gustatory/olfactory/tactile information by other senses

17. Synaesthesia

(Greek 'syn' – 'together' and 'aisthesis' – 'perception') or 'joint sensation' or 'cross-sensory perception' is an involuntary physical experience of a cross-modal association, i.e. the stimulation of one sensory modality triggers a perception in one or more different senses.

Synaesthesia can be of two types:

1. *Two-sensory synaesthesia,* when stimulation of one modality triggers the perception in a second modality, in the absence of direct stimulation of this second modality. The examples of this type are:
   - coloured-hearing or chromaesthesia: when a sound triggers the perception of a colour;
   - coloured-olfaction: when a smell triggers the perception of a colour;
   - coloured-gustation: when a taste triggers the perception of a colour;
   - tactile-gustation: when a taste is experienced as a shape;
   - audiomotor: when the sounds of different words trigger different postures or movements of the body; etc.
2. *Multiple sensory synaesthesia:*
   - coloured-numbers: when numbers are heard or read they are experienced as colours;
   - coloured-letters: when letters are heard or read they are experienced as colours;
   - coloured-graphemes: when words are heard or read they are experienced as colours;
   - shaped-numbers: when numbers are heard or read they are experienced as shapes.

In synaesthesia there can be 30 possibilities of different combinations of senses, but usually two senses cross that makes ten possible synaesthetic pairings. Some synaesthetes smell sights or taste shapes, others see sounds. Practically every combination has been reported.

More often synaesthesia is unidirectional, i.e., for example, sight may be experienced as touch but touch does not trigger visual perceptions.

One in every 25,000 people is reported to have synaesthesia (Cytowic, 1989), but this estimate might be far too low. Women synaesthetes predominate: a ratio is reported from 3:1 (Cytowic, 1989) to 8:1 (Baron-Cohen et al., 1993). Synaesthesia appears more frequently among left-handed people and is believed to be genetic. 15% of people with synaesthesia are reported to have a history of someone in their first-degree relatives having dyslexia, autism or ADD (Cytowic, 1995). Synaesthetic experience is very individual, for example, among people who see coloured sounds there is no specific colour for each sound from person to person. Learning disabilities seem more common in synaesthetes, however, the actual incidence of autism among synaesthetes is not known at present.

Cytowic (1995) defines the following five diagnostic features of synaesthesia:

1. Synaesthesia is involuntary. It is a passive experience that happens to someone. The sensations cannot be suppressed or incurred, though the intensity is influenced by the situation they occur in.
2. Synaesthesia is projected into the environment: it is not just in the head but the individual actually sees a sound, hears a sight, etc; it is perceived externally in peri-personal space, the limb-axis space immediately surrounding the body.
3. Synaesthetic perceptions are durable and generic, i.e. they do not change over time or situation and they are always experienced with the stimulus.
4. Synaesthesia is memorable: the synaethetic sensations are remembered best.
5. Synaesthesia is emotional: having this experience causes ecstasy.

One of the most common features of synaesthetes is their superior memory (due to their parallel sensations). They remember conversations, verbal instructions, spatial location of objects, etc. in every detail. Perhaps related to this is a tendency displayed by synaesthetes to prefer order, neatness, symmetry and balance. They usually perform in the superior range of the Wechsler Memory Scale (Cytowic, 1995).

Synaesthetes are observed to have uneven cognitive skills. Among their deficiencies the most commonly reported are: right-left confusion (allochiria), poor math skills and a poor sense of direction. Here we can see some similarity between the synaesthetic and autistic features. In some autistic individuals their resistance to changes, insistence on order and routine, echolalia (triggered by some stimuli), an exceptional memory for details, a poor sense of direction, etc. might be caused by synaesthesia.

There are several theories concerning the origin of synaesthesia. The most recent one is the Neonatal Synaesthesia (NS) hypothesis proposed by Maurer (1993). The author states that all human babies (neonates) have synaesthesia, i.e. experience undifferentiated sensory input, probably up to about 4 months of age. This hypothesis refutes Piaget's developmental theory (1952) that the different sensory systems are independent at birth and only gradually become integrated with one another.

Maurer's hypothesis needs more evidence to be proven. However, there are some indirect data that support his idea, e.g., neonates of other species (kittens, hamsters, etc.) have similar transient connections between visual, auditory, somatosensory and motorcortex (Dehay et al., 1984). Maurer (1993) suggests the same could be true of human babies. Some autistic people also believe that synaesthesia is an earlier phase of development of sensory systems: it "comes from a time before fixed sensory integration, before taste was taste and smell was smell, sound was sound, touch was touch and vision was vision" (Williams, 1998, 127).

If, according to the NS theory, synaesthesia is a normal phase of development, then adult synaesthesia, as was suggested by Baron-Cohen et al. (1993) might represent a breakdown in the process of modularization. Thus, the following an early initial phase of normal synaesthesia, a different (adult-like) pattern of the differentiation of the perceptual system is developed because of the development of more rapid and efficient information processing and adult synaesthesia, therefore, represents a failure to develop differentiation of the senses.

We can draw a parallel. In autism there are some phases of development that do not follow a common path. For example, infantile reflexes that are meant to become inhibited naturally in early infancy through feedback to the brain regarding changes in growth and adaptations to the environment, sometimes fail to be replaced by more functional ones and are still present in autistic adults (Williams, 1996). Probably, synaesthesia in autism is another 'remnant' that fails to become inhibited.

Most people with synaesthesia do not complain of their condition because for them it is their normal perception of the world and they are not aware of it causing any disadvantages. This leads to the paradoxical conclusion that dysmodularity is not always maladaptive (Baron-Cohen, 1996). Though it is true only if synaesthesia is unidirectional, whereas in case of 'two-ways' synaesthesia, when, for example, a synaesthete not only sees colours when he hears sounds, but also hears sounds whenever he sees colours, the individual really suffers from the condition. Baron-Cohen (1996) enumerates possible ill-effects of this type of synaesthesia: stress, dizziness, information overload, avoidance of noisy or colourful places, that lead to social withdrawal and interference with ordinary life.

Though the fact that synaesthesia does occur in autism is recognised, it is considered to be rare (Cesaroni & Garber, 1991). Probably, reported low incidence of synaesthesia in autism can be accounted for the fact that it is not easily detected in the autistic population. There are two reasons for this:

- Communication problems: even verbal individuals have difficulties in expressing their experiences;
- Even non-autistic synaesthetes find it difficult to realise that they experience the world differently and it might be hard for them to imagine that others cannot, for example, hear sounds while seeing colours. It is we who must find out whether they experience synaesthesia.

The analysis of the personal accounts of autistic individuals shows that synaesthesia is not rare in this population and practically all combinations of senses have been found. The analysis shows that such senses as sight, sound and touch are involved more often than smell and taste.

Below are the descriptions of the experiences which can be defined as synaesthetic:

Tactile-hearing:

"I loved the way most words play or ie words) hurt my ears" (Willey, 1999, 20)

"...words that tickled, words that w... oke them...(some voices, especially with heavy nasal or high shrill qu...ities, or extreme eastern or southern accents) sting my ears like a wet towel slapped against my eardrum would" (Willey, 1999, 31)

Tactile-visual:

"I would refuse words that looked ugly by virtue of being too lopsided or too cumbersome or too unusual in their phonetics" (Willey, 1999, 20).

"I knew I had written something great when I found words that looked, sounded or felt good" (Willey, 1999, 31)

Olfactory-visual:

"It is possible... not only to see colours, but almost to smell them, too" (O'Neill, 1999, 29)

Gustatory-olfactory:

(as a reaction to the perfume) "my mouth tasted like I had eaten a bunch of sickly smelling flowers" (Williams, 1999, 57)

One individual with autism (cited in Cesaroni & Garber, 1991) describes the experience of sounds as "vague sensations of colour, shape, texture, movement, scent or flavour. It is as if information was received in several modes even though the signal comes from one source". Jim Sinclair (1998) speaks about the colours of voices and the tactility of music. Donna Williams (1996) experiences some people ("fluffy people") "causing her lemons" because "it triggers a sensation that feels exactly how eating lemons" makes her feel:

"Though the taste isn't there, the response in my mouth and neck and muscles is the same. These people cause a 'sour taste' that is as extreme and of the same type that lemons cause me when eaten" (p. 90)

What to look for:

Vision:

1). Covers/rubs/hits/blinks eyes in response to a sound/taste/smell/touch.

2). Complains about (is frustrated with) the 'wrong' colours of letters/numbers, etc. written on coloured blocks, etc.

Hearing:

1). Covers/hits ears in response to a visual stimulus/taste/smell/touch/texture.

2). Complains about (is frustrated with) a sound in response to colours/textures/scent/flavour/touch.

Taste:

1). Makes swallowing movements in response to a visual/auditory stimulus/smell/touch.

2). Complains about (is frustrated with) taste in response to a visual/auditory stimulus/smell touch.

Smell:

1). Covers/rubs/hits, etc. the nose in response to a visual/auditory stimulus/taste/touch.

Tactility:

1). Complains about (is frustrated with) feeling colours/sounds, etc. while being touched.

2). Complains about (is frustrated with) feeling being touched when being looked at.

3). Complains about (is frustrated with) backache, etc./heat/cold in colourful/crowded, etc. places with lots of movement.

4). Involuntary movements/postures of the body in response to a visual/auditory stimulus/smell/taste.

18. Perceptual memory ("sense memory" – Donna Williams)

Many autistic people have a very good perceptual memory, especially a visual memory for details that others miss (O'Neill, 1999).

Some people claim that their earliest memories are from a period of just a few months old and even prior to their birth when they recall being able to hear their mother's heartbeat (Cesaroni & Garber, 1991; Walker & Cantello, 1994).

Many people with autism remember not verbally but while remembering they see, hear, feel, taste the items. For example, Willey (1999) reports about her 'tactile memories':

> *"I can still feel what it was like to open books so wide their covers touched back to back. I remember the way the book would resist my forcing it to open that far-reaching" (p. 16)*

Any time she even thought about textures she hates, goose bumps and chills and a general sense of unease would follow (Willey, 1999, 22).

The most commonly reported are the feats of visual and auditory memory. Well-known pictures of Stephen Wiltshire, an autistic savant, of architectural buildings contain the smallest details such as style and size of windows, and this is despite the fact that he saw the original buildings only once for a few minutes and did not begin his drawings immediately. It is the so-called eidetic or photographic memory, which allows these people to create visualisations that are so intense as those brought about the original stimuli (Carter, 1998).

Some researchers (Rose, 1993) suggest that up to 50% of 5-year-olds have the ability to 'see' an imagined image as though it was really there. Some adults are reported to retain this ability (see, e.g., Schatzman, 1980).

Clara Park (1967) says that her autistic daughter's eye is like a camera: she draws pictures of houses very accurately, with finest detail. Temple Grandin (1996a) writes about Barbara, a woman with autism, whose ability to recognise pattern, has made her one of the best technicians in the laboratory identifying cancer cells. Her visual abilities enable her to spot abnormal cells instantly, because they "just jump out at her".

Some autistic individuals are reported (O'Neill, 1999) to be able to spell excellently thanks to their visual/photographic memory: as they read they quickly memorise the spellings of words; when they misspell a word they can refer to their mental catalogue of data to recall which spelling looks more accurate. Temple Grandin (1996a) describes her process of remembering things as follows: "I store information in my head as if it were on a CD-ROM disc. When I recall something I have learned, I replay the video in my imagination" (p. 24). Her memory patterns are similar to those described by A.R.Luria (1987) who studied a man with amazing feats of memory: when the man heard or read a word, it was at once converted into a visual image corresponding with the object of the word signified for him.

Recent research (Welling, 1994) shows that the ability to rapidly identify all the prime numbers in a list of numbers by mathematically weak autistic individuals could be based on their visual memory: they visually analyse the symmetry of numbers, that enables them to distinguish prime from nonprime numbers.

Some autistic people, while having excellent recall memory (photographic memory), have problems with recognition memory, for example, Jared Blackburn has trouble recognising faces, letters, etc. without actively visualising them (Blackburn, 1999). Some autistic people have a very good auditory memory ('sound memory, 'audiographic memory' – Williams, 1996), that enables them to repeat ('replay') long strings of things they have heard. Some can record musical pieces in their minds, then hum or play them flawlessly on an instrument later on (O'Neill, 1999). Some can 'hear' conversations in their memory (Willey, 1999), etc. It is like replaying a tape recording of conversations, songs heard and so on. (Williams, 1998, 127).

What to look for:

Displays a good visual/auditory/gustatory/olfactory/tactile memory.

19. "Serial memory" (Williams) is a type of associative memory, triggered by sensory stimuli.

Donna Williams (1994) describes it as follows:

> *"I used to delight in my memory, which was acute sometimes perfect to the finest detail. I could set off one part of it and run like a serial as I described the pictures, became the narrator of a silent movie, the verbal animator of a recorded soundtrack"* (p. 48)

Serial memories can be triggered by smells, by a certain colour or pattern, by a sequence of words, by a particular physical action, by touch, etc. (Williams, 1996, 194). For example, the word "under" triggered Temple Grandin to picture herself getting under the cafeteria tables at school during an air-raid drill, then she continued to 'play video' of the teacher scolding her after she hit Alfred for putting dirt on her shoe, and then 'saw' submarines under the Antarctic and the Beatles song "Yellow Submarine"; if she let her mind pause on the picture of the yellow submarine, she then heard the song; then she would start humming the song and get to the part about people coming on board, and her association would switch to the gangway of a ship she had seen in Australia, etc. (1996a, 30).

Seeing the black and white stripes on a toy plane can trigger the memory of eating humbugs in a classroom many years before and might run into who was in the class on that day and what was being taught and the noise that the book made when snapped closed and the exact path the teacher travelled across the room at a particular point, etc, etc. (Williams, 1996, 194). Touching the doorway to a room may trigger the serial memory of touching the same door of the same room another time and the events that happened after this (Williams, 1996, 148).

Many autistic children use the serial memory as a compensation for their inability to process information quickly (delayed processing): they do not process information at the time it happens, they respond to the situation 'from memory' when something remembered in a serial way is triggered. They often cannot keep track of conversation as in the short break between two halves of a sentence, there may have been triggered a huge number of tracks, leading to tracks, leading to tracks (Williams, 1996). They just cannot stop endless associations (Grandin, 1996a, 25).

What to look for:

1). Reactions are triggered by some stimuli.

2). Uses songs, commercials, etc. to respond

3). Uses idiosyncratic routinised responses

4). Cannot keep track of conversation

20. Perceptual thinking.

There appear to be two basic types of thinking in autistic people: totally perceptual (usually visual) thinkers and the music, math and memory thinkers (Grandin, 1999).

One of the characteristics of autism is the remarkable ability of most autistic people to excel at visual-spatial skills while performing very poorly at verbal skills. For those who have visual thinking ("thinking in pictures" – Grandin), words are like a second language; their thought processes are different from language-based thinkers. Temple Grandin describes this as follows:

> *"I translate both spoken and written words into full-color movies, complete with sound, which run like a VCR tape in my head. When somebody speaks to me, his words are instantly translated into pictures. Language-based thinkers often find this phenomenon difficult to understand, but in my job as an equipment designer for the livestock industry, visual thinking is a tremendous advantage. Visual thinking has enabled me to build entire systems in my imagination" (1996a, 19)*

Recent research findings (Farah, 1989; Zeki, 1992) show that verbal thought and visual thinking work via different brain systems. These studies reveal that in brain-damaged patients one system can be damaged, while another system may be normal. In autism, the systems that process visual-spatial information are intact (Grandin, 1996b).

Many people with autism are reported to 'think in pictures' or 'in sounds'. Temple Grandin describes an autistic composer who made 'sound pictures' and an autistic computer programmer who visualised the entire programme tree in his mind and then filled in the programme code on each branch (1996b)

Most of Jared Blackburn's thinking (reasoning, planning) is visual:

> *"Ideas come to me as images, and I can take things apart and put them together in my imagination very well; I used to design machines… completely in my imagination. I can plan paintings or room design in my head, and can manipulate images to solve most problems. I can often measure objects by visualizing a ruler (etc.) moving along the object" (1999, 11)*

Not all people with autism are highly visual thinkers. They appear to be on a continuum of visualisation skills ranging from next to none, to seeing vague generalised pictures, to seeing semi-specific pictures, to seeing, as in the case of Temple Grandin, in very specific pictures (Grandin, 1996a, 28). Unlike most people who think from general to specific, 'visual thinkers' move from video-like, specific images to generalisation and concepts, for example:

> *"…my concept of dogs is inextricably linked to every dog I've ever known. It's as if I have a card catalogue of dogs I have seen, complete with pictures which continually grows as I add more examples to my video library" (Grandin, 1996a, 28)*

When Temple Grandin designs work, she can "test run" the equipment in her imagination (Grandin, 1999, 4). 'Visual thinkers' often have difficulty with long verbal information, and prefer written texts:

> *"When I read, I translate written words into color movies or simply store a photo of the written page to be read later. When I retrieve the material I see a photocopy of the page in my imagination" (Grandin, 1996a, 31)*

For Donna Williams, not being able to visualise quickly something described to her, or mentally hold visualisation together well in any continuous or detailed way, means that verbal descriptions are very hard to make much sense of. For her, having trouble visualising also means that it is very hard to alter a mental image once she has achieved one, so the effect of new information in altering old information does not happen so smoothly (Williams, 1996, 166).

Autistic people often have problems learning abstract things that cannot be thought about in pictures. To understand abstract concepts they use visual images. For example:

> *"I thought of peace as a dove, an Indian peace pipe... Honesty was represented by an image of placing one's hand on the Bible in court..." (Grandin, 1996a, 33)*

To understand personal relationships some autistic individuals used the image of sliding doors (Grandin, 1996a,b).

Autistic children usually learn nouns first as nouns are easily associated with pictures in their mind. Words that have no concrete visual meaning, such as 'put', or 'on', or 'over', have no meaning for them until they have a visual image to fix them in the memory (Grandin, 1996a,b; Park, 1967). For example, Donna Williams became frustrated when she could not find an 'of' button on her calculator to find percents. To understand verbs and adverbs Temple Grandin has learned to visualise them:

> *"The word 'jumping' triggered a memory of jumping hurdles at the mock Olympics held at my elementary school. Adverbs often trigger inappropriate images – 'quickly' reminds me of Nestle's Quik – unless they are paired with a verb, which modifies my visual image... As a child, I left out words such as 'is', 'the', and 'it', because they had no meaning by themselves. Similarly, words like 'of' and 'an' made no sense... To this day certain verb conjugations, such as 'to be', are absolutely meaningless to me" (Grandin, 1996a, 30, 31)*

Visual thinking can account for some other language idiosyncrasies, observed by Frith (1989), such as, that an autistic child may say "French toast" when he is happy, etc.

Visual thinking is often associated with intellectual giftedness. Albert Einstein, for example, was a visual thinker who failed his high school language exam and relied on visual methods of study (Holton, 1971-1972). He developed the theory of relativity by imagining himself on a beam of light (Patten, 1973). Unlike Temple Grandin, he could decode his visual images into mathematical formulas; i.e. he could connect visual and mathematical thinking.

The examples of gustatory and olfactory images can be 'gustatory/olfactory hallucinations', reported by some autistic people.

What to look for:

1). Easily solves jigsaw puzzles

2). Remembers the routes and places

3). Memorises enormous amounts of information at a glance

4). Poor at mathematics

5). Learns nouns first

6). Has difficulties with adverbs and prepositions

7). Idiosyncratic patterns in language development, e.g., names one thing to denote the other, etc.

All the patterns are summarised in the table.

Possible Patterns of Sensory Experiences in Autism

	Vision	Hearing	Tactility	Taste	Smell
1. Intensity the senses work	Hyper-, hypo-	Hyper-, hypo-	Hyper-, hypo-	Hyper-, hypo	Hyper-, hypo-
2. Inconsistency of perception	Fluctuation between hyper -& hypo; 'in' – 'out'	Fluctuation between hyper- & hypo-; 'in' – 'out'	Fluctuation between Hyper- & hypo-; 'in' – 'out'	Fluctuation between hyper- & hypo-	Fluctuation between hyper- & hypo-
3. 'Mono'-processing (number of channels working at a time)	Shutting down other channels while seeing	Shutting down other channels while hearing	Shutting down other channels while touching or being touched	Shutting down other channels while tasting	Shutting down other channels while smelling
4. Fragmented perception. Partial Perception	Seeing 'in bits'. Prosopagnosia	Hearing 'in bits'	Feeling touch, cold/hot 'in bits'	Tasting 'in bits'	Smelling 'in bits'
5. Distorted perception	Poor/distorted depth & space perception; seeing 2D world; distortions of shape, size, etc.	Hearing sounds or intonation rather than words; distorted sound, etc.	Distorted tactile perception	Distorted gustatory perception	Distorted olfactory perception
6. Peripheral perception. Avoidance of central/ direct perception	Peripheral vision. Avoidance of eye contact	Hearing if listening to somebody indirectly	Peripheral tactile perception	Peripheral gustatory perception	Peripheral olfactory perception
7. Inability to (distinguish between) filter foreground and background	'Optical disillusions', inability to filter visual stimuli	Inability to screen out background noise	Inability to distinguish between tactile stimuli of different Intensity	Inability to distinguish between strong & weak tastes	Inability to distinguish between strong & weak smell
8. Sensitivity to (disturbance by) some stimuli	Light/colour sensitivity. Disturbance by some patterns	Disturbance by some sounds	Sensitivity to certain textures	Disturbance by some gustatory stimuli	Disturbance by some olfactory stimuli
9. Fascination with certain stimuli	Fascination with patterns, lights, colours, etc.	Fascination with sounds	Fascination with tactile stimuli	Fascination with certain flavours	Fascination with certain smells

Possible patterns of sensory experiences in autism. continued

10.'Losing oneself' in certain stimuli. Resonance	Merging/ getting in resonance with lights, colours, patterns	Merging/ getting in resonance with sounds	Merging/ getting in resonance with tactile stimuli; feeling pain of other people	Merging/ getting in resonance with tastes	Merging/ getting in resonance with smells
11Daydreaming	'Seeing' thoughts, emotions of other people; events that don't relate to oneself	'Hearing' thoughts of other people; events	'Feeling' events	'Gustatory hallucinations'	'Olfactory hallucinations'
12.Delayed perception	Delayed processing of visual stimuli	Delayed processing of auditory stimuli	Delayed processing of tactile stimuli	Delayed processing of tastes	Delayed processing of smells
13.Vulnerability to sensory overload	Light refraction ('shine') etc.	Sound overload ('sound reverberation')	Tactile overload	Gustatory overload	Olfactory overload
14.Systems shutdowns	Visual 'whiteouts'. 'White darkness'	Auditory 'tuneouts'. 'Loud silence'	Tactile 'tuneouts'	Gustatory 'tuneouts'	Olfactory 'tuneouts'
15.'Sensory agnosia' (difficulty interpreting a sense)	'Meaning-blindness'. Feeling/acting 'blind'	'Meaning-deafness'. Feeling/acting 'deaf'	'Touch deadness'	Difficulty interpreting tastes	Difficulty interpreting smells
16.Compensating for unreliable sense by other senses	Testing visual perception perception by other senses	Testing auditory perception by other senses	Testing tactile perception by other senses	Testing gustatory perception by other senses	Testing olfactory perception by other senses
17.Synaesthesia	Seeing sounds, smells, temperature, etc.	Hearing colours, flavours, touch, etc.	When being touched feeling colours, etc.	Tasting colours, sounds, etc.	Smelling sounds, colours, etc.
18.Perceptual memory	Visual ('photographic') memory	'Audiographic/ sound memory'	Tactile memory	Gustatory memory	Olfactory memory
19.'Serial memory'	Triggered by visual stimuli	Triggered by auditory stimuli	Triggered by tactile stimuli	Triggered by tastes, flavours	Triggered by smells
20.Perceptual thinking	Visual thinking ('Thinking in pictures')	'Auditory pictures'	'Tactile images'	'Gustatory images'	'Olfactory images'

Chapter 3

"RAINBOWS"

All the findings from the personal accounts have been organized into a screening tool for compiling a Sensory Profile Checklist (SPC, Appendix 1). This checklist is completed by the parents of the child. However, while the input from the parents is very important, particularly regarding the child's sensory history and behaviour at home, it is also necessary to observe the child during sessions at school or at the clinic in order to consolidate the parental information and check some points marked in the SPC as "not sure". The observation is conducted in the form of 'incident' sampling – each time the target behaviour occurs a box is ticked. To organize and summarize the observations Observation Checklists prove to be very useful. They include a list of behaviours (sensorisms) which should be checked for the child. At the stage of interpretations of the findings the parents and the children should be actively involved. The discussions with the parents are vital as they help not only to compile the SPC for their child but also to understand the child's behaviours. The children should be encouraged to analyze their own behaviours and give their own interpretation of them through verbal explanation and/or drawings (how they feel and perceive the world).

The data obtained from this can be presented in the form of specially worked out graphs - "rainbows" with the boxes, representing specific features experienced by the individuals, coloured in. The numbers in the graph coincide with the characteristics enumerated in the table. Different colours can be used for each sensory channel: e.g. red – for vision, orange – for hearing, yellow – for tactility, green – for taste, blue – for smell. The extent to which each channel is affected is demonstrated when the "rainbows" are coloured in as the number of coloured sections corresponds to the number of characteristics experienced by the individual.

The reason the symbol of a rainbow was chosen to indicate probable sensory experiences was that many autistic people compare autism with a rainbow and describe autistic world as a rainbow prism (Blackburn, 1997; O'Neill, 1999). Besides, it seems appropriate to show sensory profile of an autistic individual in the form of curved lines rather than a straight line, as not all sensory differences are deficits, some are better described as superabilities (or gifts) that could be successfully used in the treatment of autistic people. Figures 1-4 show the "rainbows" compiled for four children diagnosed as having autism. The graphs reveal the diversity of sensory problems experienced by each child, while the symptoms 'on the surface' (DSM-IV, ICD-10) are the same.

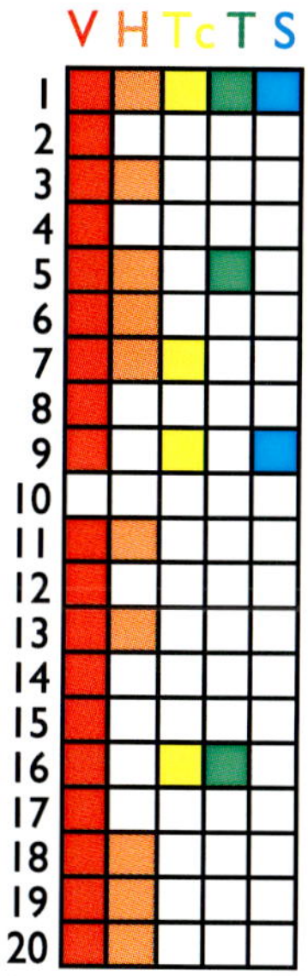

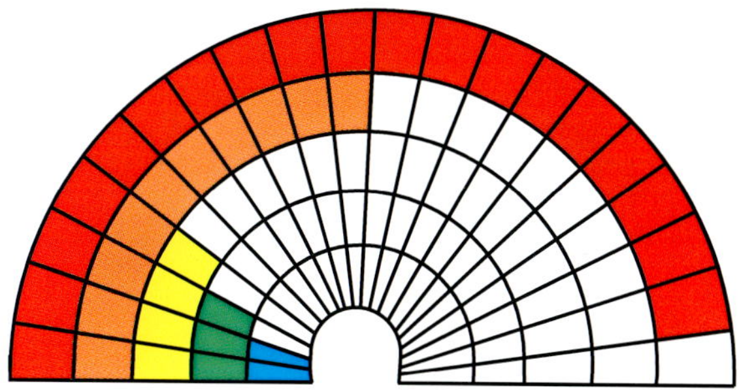

Figure 1. Alex's Rainbow

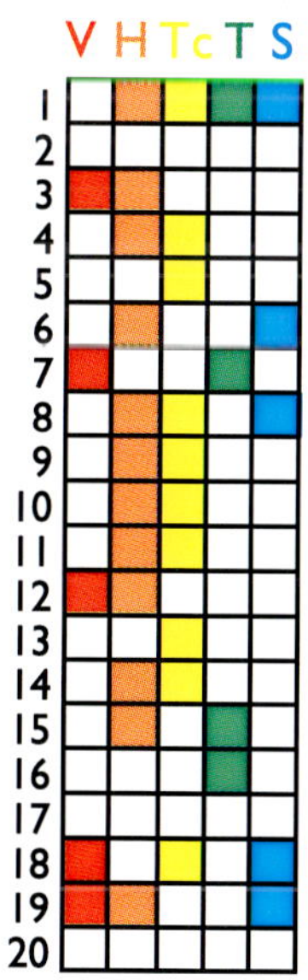

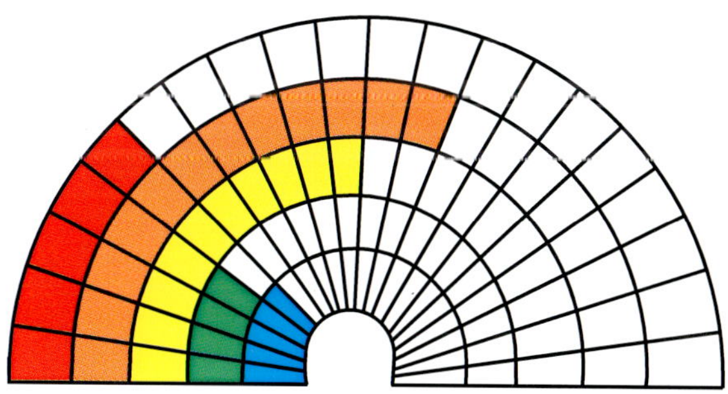

Figure 1. Vicky's Rainbow

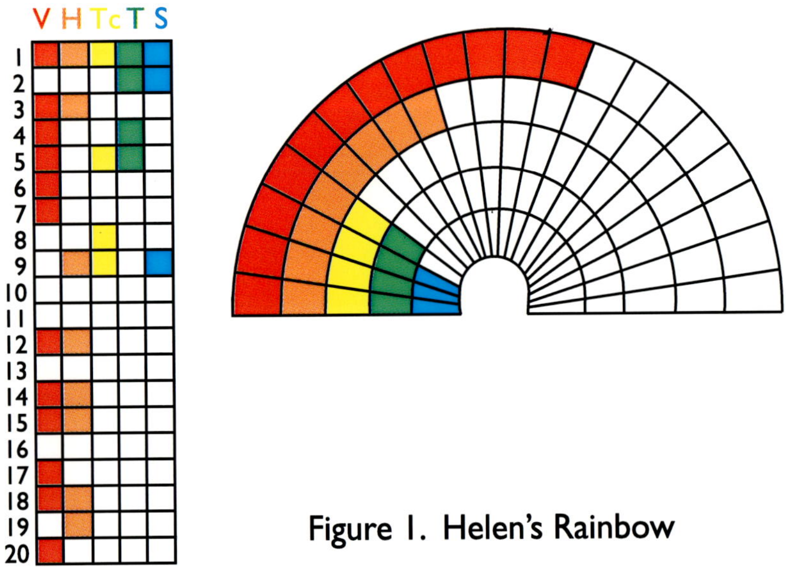

Figure 1. Helen's Rainbow

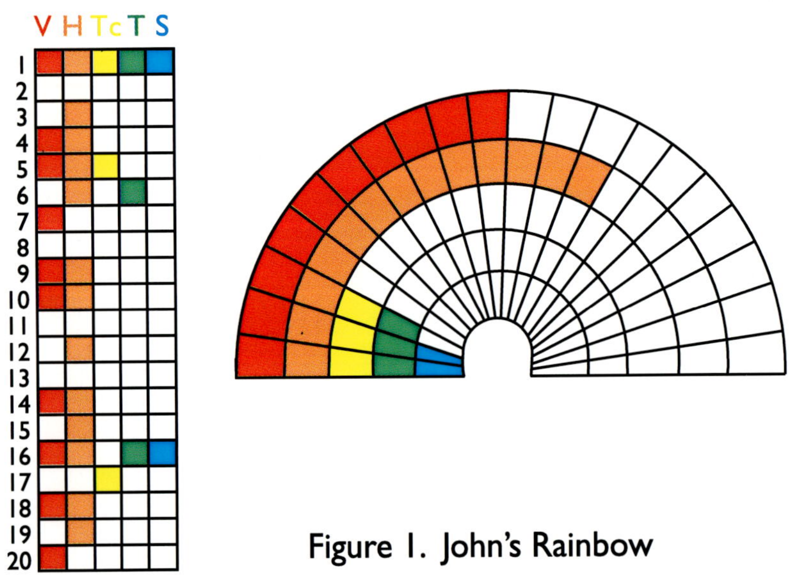

Figure 1. John's Rainbow

Chapter 4

CASE STUDIES

Background information about the children:

(The names of the children have been changed)

Alex is an 11-year-old boy, diagnosed as autistic at the age of 5. At the age of 8 he was also diagnosed as suffering from Scotopic Sensitivity/Irlen Syndrome. Alex started talking at the age of 6, now he still has articulation difficulties. His receptive language is fairly good, his expressive language is limited to short statements and questions and is often idiosyncratic, though he is generally able to communicate his wants and needs.

Alex's primary problem at the moment is his aggressive behaviour.

Helen is a 7-year-old girl, diagnosed as autistic at the age of 6, verbal (started talking at the age of 3), echolalic.

The girl is hyperactive, often does not react to the instructions, socially withdrawn.

John is an 11-year-old boy, diagnosed as autistic at the age of 2, verbal, though both receptive and expressive language is limited, echolalic. The boy is often withdrawn, passive, displays mild learning difficulties.

Vicky is a 14-year-old girl, diagnosed as autistic at the age of 7, verbal, has articulation difficulties. Both receptive and expressive language is fairly good. Vicky has mild learning difficulties.

The primary problem at the moment is her self-injurious behaviour.

Below are some of the summarized data of the observations:

1. Intensity (hyper-, hypo-):

Alex's vision is very acute (hyper): he could see the tiniest particles in the air, describing them as "moths": "Moths are flying". He notices every tiny change in the environment: "The rubber is under the teacher's table" "The picture is not straight", etc. He hates bright lights and is frightened by lightning.

Helen's vision is hypo: she is attracted by any shining object, looks intensely at people, and is fascinated with mirrors. At the lesson she could move fingers in front of her face for hours.

Vicky's and Alex's hearing is very acute. They can hear what is going on in the next room but one: "The chair is being moved. The ruler has been dropped", etc.

Helen's hearing is hypo: She enjoys banging doors, cannot tolerate silence, and if there is not enough noise for her, she produces sounds herself.

John (hypoauditory) likes any sound: running water, traffic, crowds.

Vicky cannot tolerate any touch, while Helen likes pressure, rough game.

Vicky's sense of smell is hyper: if she is being touched by somebody, she immediately smells the place of touch, and more often than not she takes off her jacket or dress with this 'spoilt spot' and refuses to wear it again unless it is washed.

2. Inconsistency of perception:

Alex can respond differently to the same visual (colours, patterns) or auditory (the sound of heating system, fan) stimuli depending on his physical state and the value of his "cup" (See 13. 'Vulnerability to overload' in the analysis)

Helen can eat her favorite food (sausage) on one day and refuse even to approach it on the other.

3. Mono-processing:

If John is looking at something (e.g., the teacher is showing the card with number 10), he does not hear the instruction ("Say the previous number") and seems very confused without any knowledge of what is expected of him.

4. Fragmented perception:

Vicky's often has problems with parts of her clothes: "It hurts here" (trying to tear off her right sleeve while ignoring her left one), or "My back is hot".

Alex's "seeing in bits": "Her leg disturbs me". "Dasha's (the cat) head has turned round".

5. Distorted perception:

Helen does not seem to feel the boundaries of her body and its position in the classroom. She often hits herself when confused with the instruction, e.g.: "Don't lean over the table".

Vicky has poor depth and space perception. She is afraid of descending the stairs, and when ascending she lifts her feet too high above the stair.

Alex's perception of people and himself is distorted. The distortions depend on the state he is in. E.g., when asked to draw himself he could give different versions: Fig. 5 "Self-portrait" when he was relaxed; Fig. 6 "Self-portrait" when he was irritated with the task. After an outburst of aggression he was invited to draw a picture "Alex in panic" (Fig. 7). During the discussion about the origin of "his panic" he was asked to show the "panic" on the picture, and he drew himself with an arrow pointing at his head ("panic") and said: "I had a headache and the eyes misbehaved".

Figures 5 "Self Portrait" (1)

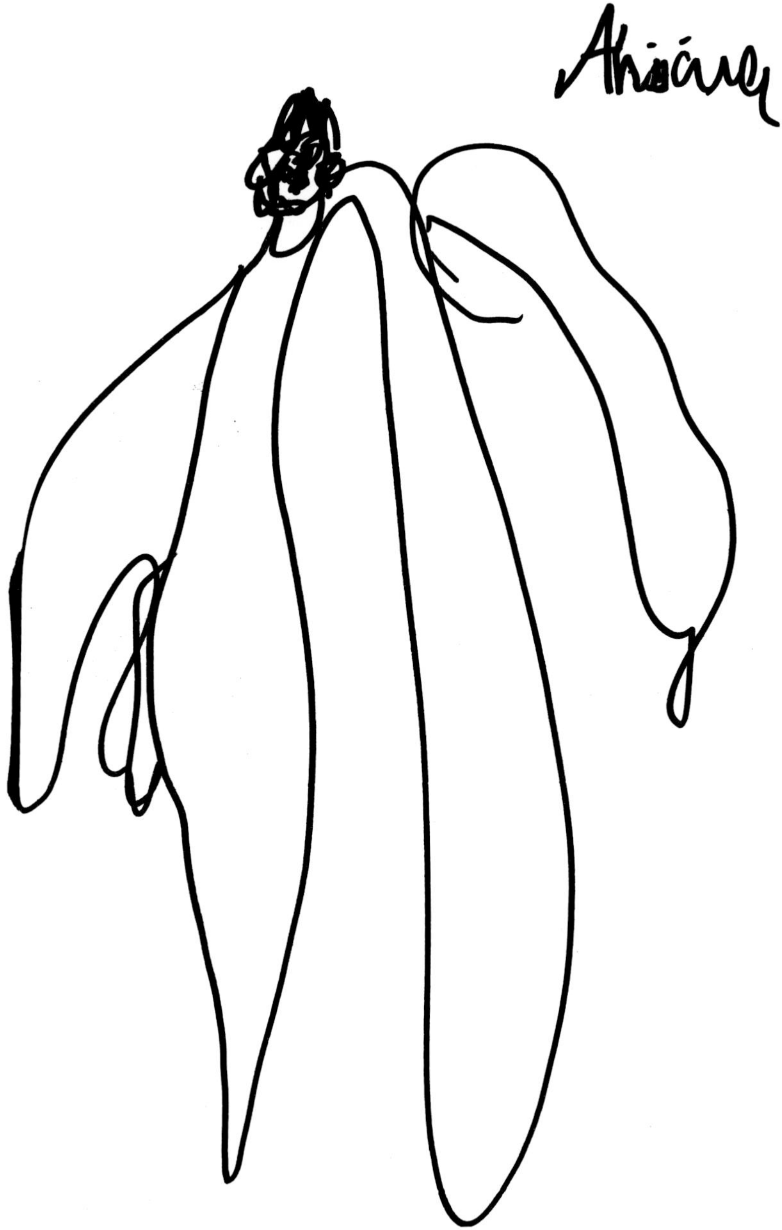

Figures 6 "Self Portrait" (2)

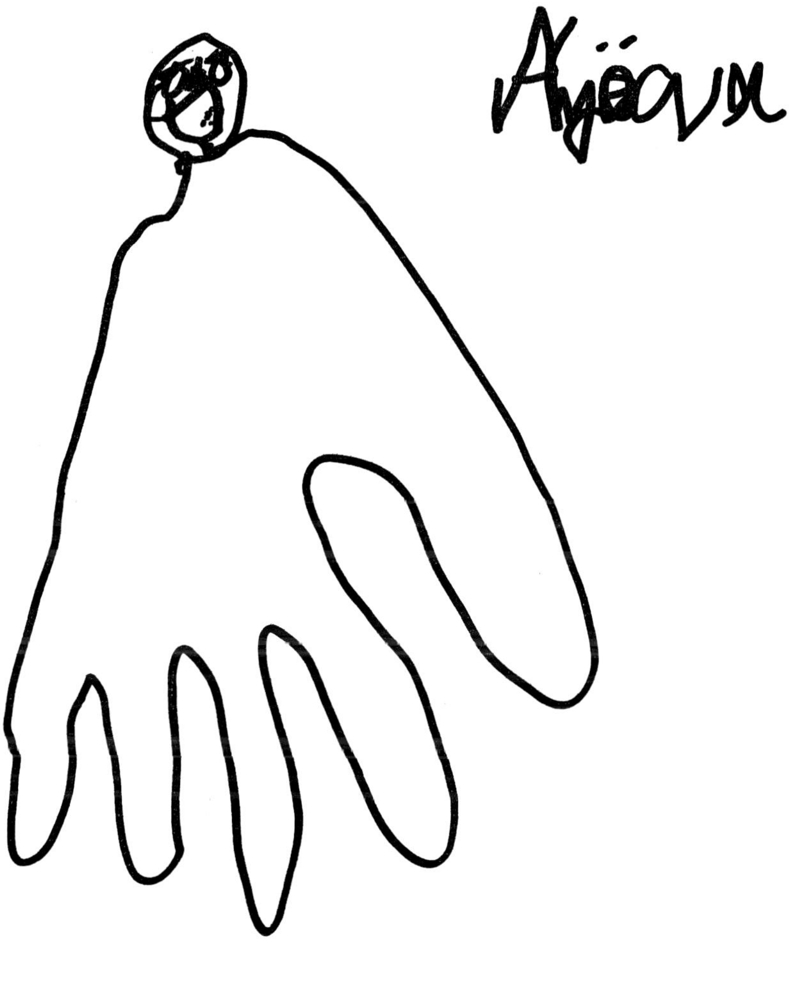

Figures 7 "A. in panic" (Location of panic is shown with an arrow)

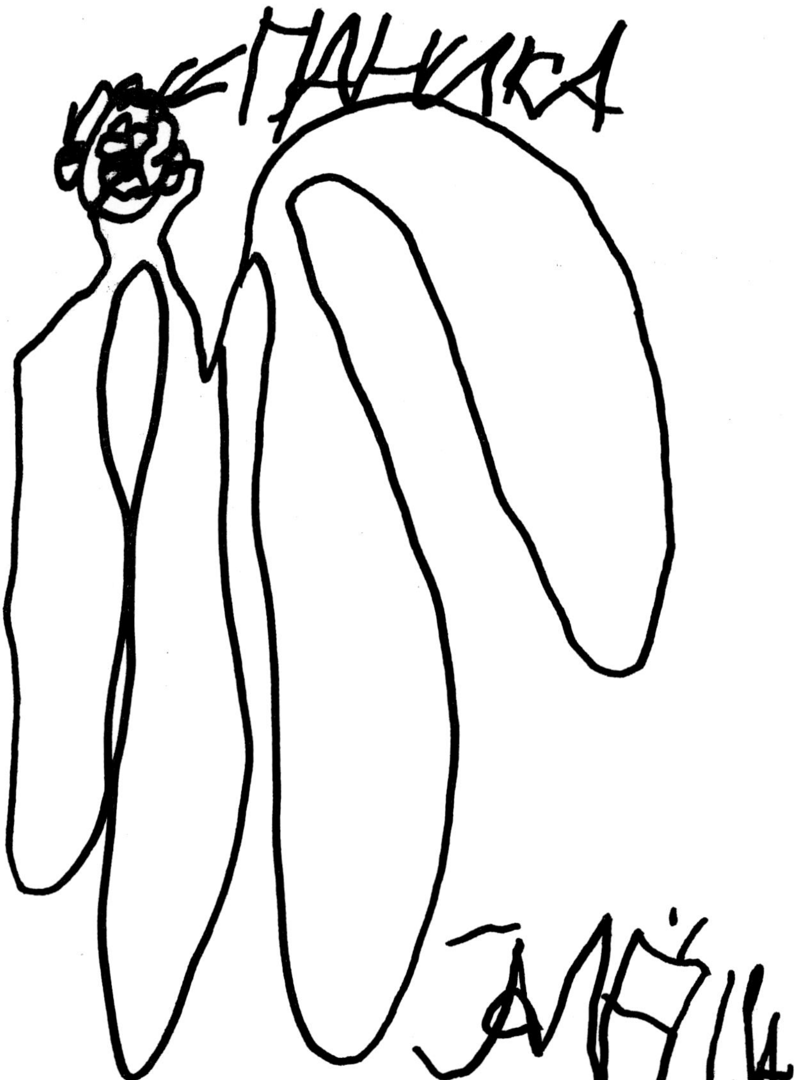

6. Peripheral perception. Avoidance of central/direct perception:

Alex, John and Vicky 'hear better' (i.e. react to the instructions) if the instructions are 'addressed to the wall'. Alex and Helen often use their peripheral vision and seem to see what is going on without direct looking at it. Alex cannot tolerate when someone is looking at him directly and makes them turn away ("Don't look", "Turn away"). He even complains if the cat is looking at him.

7. Inability to distinguish between foreground and background:

The children were not fooled by optical illusions and gave a very quick answer when asked what they saw in the typical pictures of optical illusions ("A vase and two faces", etc.) Alex and Vicky display the same feature in hearing: they could not concentrate on the verbally given task while heating was working, and they were more interested in other sound and were trying to find the source of them.

8., 9. Sensitivity to (disturbance by) some stimuli. Fascination with certain stimuli.

One and the same stimulus can cause disturbance and fascination to different children. For example, Vicky hates the sound of running water, whereas John is fascinated with it. Alex is disturbed by bright lights, whereas Helen is enjoying looking at them.

10. "Losing oneself" in certain stimuli. 'Resonance':

John seems to be absorbed with colours and sounds, and can 'lose himself' in them, if not interrupted.

11. Daydreaming:

As the expressive language of the children is limited, it is difficult to say whether they experience this. Though, sometimes, Vicky's mother "feels" she "reads" her emotions, no matter how hard she tries to hide them.

12. Delayed perception:

All the children display delayed perception to the auditory stimuli: they can respond to the question in a few minutes (John, Helen and Vicky) or even in a few days (Alex).

13. Vulnerability to sensory overload:

Alex is very vulnerable to sensory overload. The speed with which his "cup has been being filled in" depends on the number and intensity of the stimuli, e.g., if there are two or more people are talking at once he is sure to be overwhelmed; or bright lights and lots of movement around him will cause his outburst in a few minutes.

14. Systems shutdowns:

Sensory overload often cause systems shutdowns when, for example, John and Helen seemed to be mindless followers without any awareness what was going on around them.

15. "Sensory agnosia":

Helen often behaves as if she were deaf: she does not react to any sound at all and does not seem to understand what the teacher asks her.

16. Compensating for unreliable sense by other senses:

John and Alex smell, touch or tap objects to check their visual perception of it. Vicky always inspects her food before eating it.

17. Synaesthesia:

Helen and Alex seem to "see" some sounds. Alex even tries to describe this experience: "I was scared. I saw a yellow 'z-z-z' sound", "The eyes saw the wrong word" (in response to a verbal instruction).

John displays involuntary movements of the body in response to some auditory stimuli (vacuum cleaners, lawn mowers).

18. Perceptual memory:

Alex, John and Helen display a very good visual and auditory memory. Vicky can distinguish the slightest difference between very similar textures.

19. "Serial Memory":

Helen can start reciting poems, triggered by one word, then jumps to the recollection of the party triggered by the word in the poem, etc. Alex and Vicky's "serial memory" can be triggered by auditory and visual stimuli.

20. Perceptual thinking:

John and Helen are very good at jigsaw puzzles. Helen, for instance, can easily solve a jigsaw puzzle of 120 pieces.

Alex, John and Helen easily memorize enormous amounts of information at a glance (though, its reproduction should be properly triggered, for example, instructions given by the same person with the same intonation, etc.).

After the analysis of the Questionnaire, observations and discussion with the parents, "rainbows" were compiled for each child (See Fig. 1-4). It turned out, despite the same diagnosis and often very similar behavioural symptoms, sensory profiles of the children were strikingly different.

CONCLUSIONS

This study attempts to define the role of sensory dysfunction in autism identified as by the sufferers themselves. It shows that sensory issues, often ignored by many professionals, are highlighted by autistic individuals in their personal accounts as one of the main problems they experience in their functioning. They claim that many behaviours, described as symptoms of autism in the diagnostic classifications, are often caused by their sensory experiences.

The analysis of the personal accounts allows us to reconstruct the sensory world of autism and to single out possible patterns of autistic people's sensory experiences. This 'inside-out' approach to the problem reveals that not all sensory experiences are dysfunctional, and some of them might be classified as 'superabilities' and considered as strengths rather than weaknesses.

All the findings from the personal accounts are classified and organized into a screening tool for compiling a Sensory Profile of an autistic child as a supplement to diagnostic classifications (DSM-IV, ICD-10) that do not include sensory characteristics.

It is very useful to 'narrow' the terms to describe different sensory perceptions. For example, the statement, "the child is hypersensitive to visual stimuli", does not say much about this particular child's visual experiences, as the child's vision might be distorted, peripheral, too acute, etc. Distinguishing between different 'hypersensitivities' allows us to address that particular child's deficits while using his strengths.

Teachers and other professionals who work with autistic children need to recognize sensory differences in autism. As the SPC can provide information about the sensory processing skills and deficiencies of autistic children, it can be used for selecting appropriate methods and planning intervention for these children.

As all the senses are integrated, the deficiency in one may lead to disturbances in the other(s). "Rainbows" are supposed to assist in finding out which sense(s) and to what extent are deficient.

Treatment programmes that are appropriate and beneficial for one child may be painful and harmful for the other. Thus, if the 'right problem' is addressed, the child gets more chances to benefit from the treatment. A widely known example of this is described by Annabel Stehli (1991) concerning her daughter Georgiana who suffered from extremely acute hearing. After the Auditory Integration Treatment her hypersensitivity to sound diminished and this enabled her to cope with other perceptual problems to such an extent that she is no longer considered autistic.

Parents often confess that what was intolerable about their child's behaviour was that it seemed meaningless. When they could understand the reason for the behaviour, it did not seem strange or disturbing any more and this led to acceptance.

This book shows the possible direction to follow in the field of sensory dysfunction in autism. Besides, it could be a starting point for selection of methods and, probably, working out new ones, in order to address the individual needs of each particular child.

REFERENCES

American Psychiatric Association (1994) *Diagnostic and Statistical Manual of Mental Disorders (DSM),* 4th ed., Washington, DC: APA

Ayres, A.J. (1979) *Sensory Integration and the Child,* Los Angeles: Western Psychological Services

Ayres, A.J. (1989) *Sensory Integration and Praxis Tests,* Los Angeles: Western Psychological Services

Baron-Cohen, S. (1996) 'Is there a normal phase of synaesthesia in Development?' *PSYCHE,* 2(27), June 1996

Baron-Cohen, S., Harrison, J., Goldstein, L., Wyke (1993) 'Coloured speech perception: Is synaesthesia what happens when modularity breaks down?' *Perception,* 22, 419-426

Baron-Cohen, S., Leslie, A.M., Frith, U. (1985) 'Does the child with autism have a theory of mind: a case specific developmental delay.' *Cognition,* 21, 37 46.

Berk, R.A., DeGangi, G.A. (1983) *DeGangi-Berk Test of Sensory Integration,* Los Angeles: Western Psychological Services

Bill (1997) Bill Choisser *Face Blind!* Bill's Face Blindness (Prosopagnosia) Pages, http://www.choisser.com/faceblind/

Bogdashina, O.B. (1999) *Autism. Part 1: Definitions and Diagnosis,* Donetsk: Lebed, (in Russian)

Carter, R. (1998) *Mapping the Mind,* London: Weidenfeld & Nicolson

Cass, H. (1996) 'Visual impairments and autism – What we know about causation and early identification', Autism and Visual Impairment Conference, *Sensory Series,* 5, 2-24

Cesaroni, L., Garber, M. (1991) 'Exploring the experiences of autism through first-hand accounts', *Journal of Autism and Developmental Disorders*, 21(3)

Cytowic, R.E. (1989) *Synaesthesia: A Union of the Senses*, New York: Springer Verlag

Cytowic, R.E. (1995) 'Synaesthesia: phenomenology and neuropsychology. A review of current knowledge', *PSYCHE*, 2(10) July 1995

Dehay, C., Bullier, J., Kennedy, H. (1984) 'Transient projections from the fronto-parietal and temporal cortex to areas 17, 18, and 19 in kitten', *Experimental Brain Research*, 57, 208-212

Delacato, C. (1974) *The Ultimate Stranger: the autistic child*, Noveto, CA: Academic Therapy Publications

Doman, R.J. (1984) *Sensory Deprivation*, NACD

Donnelly, J. (1999) *Speaking for Themselves; The Thoughts and Words of Individuals with Autism*, Autism99 Internet Conference, http://www.autism99.org/

Farah, M.J. (1989) 'The neural basis of mental imagery', *Trends in Neuroscience*, 12, 395-399

Fay, W., Schuler, A. (1980) *Emerging Language in Children with Autism*, Baltimore, MD: University Park Press

Feigenberg, I.M. (1986) *To See – to Predict – to Act*, Moscow: Znanie (in Russian)

Freeman, B.J. (1993) *Diagnosis of the Syndrome of Autism: Questions Parents Ask*, University of California

Frith, U. (1989) *Autism: Explaining the Enigma*, Oxford: Basil Blackwell

Gense, M.H., Gense, D.J. (1994) 'Identifying autism in children with blindness and visual impairment', *Review*, 26, 56-62

Gillingham, G. (1991) 'Autism: disability or superability', *Collected Papers: Therapeutic Approaches to Autism. Research and Practice*, Sunderland

Happe, F. (1994) *Autism: An Introduction to Psychological Theory*, London: UCL Press

Happe, F. (1996) 'Studying weak central coherance at low levels: Children with autism do not succumb to visual illusions: *A research note.' Journal of Child Psychology and Psychiatry*, 37, 873-877

Holton, G. (1971-1972) 'On trying to understand scientific genius', *American Scholar*, 41

Irlen, H. (1991) *Reading by the Colors: Overcoming dyslexia and other reading disabilities through the Irlen method*, New York: Avery

Jordan, R., Powell, S. (1990) *The Special Curricular Needs of Autistic Children: Learning and Thinking Skills*, The Association of Heads and Teachers of Adults and Children with Autism, London

Kanner, L. (1943) 'Autistic disturbances of affective contact', *Nervous Child*, 2, 217-250

Lovaas, O.I., Schreibman, L., Koegel, R.L., Rehm, R. (1971) 'Selective responding by autistic children to multiple sensory input', *Journal of Abnormal Psychology*, 77, 211-222

Luria, A.R. (1987) *The Mind of a Mnemonist*, Harvard University Press, Cambridge, Mass.

Maurer, D. (1993) 'Neonatal synaesthesia: implications for the processing of speech and faces', in de Boysson-Bardies, B., de Schonen, S., Jusczyk, P., McNeilage, P., Morton, J. (eds.) *Developmental Neurocognition: Speech and faces processing in the first year of life*, Kluwer Academic Publishers, Dordrecht

Ornitz, E.M. (1989) 'Autism at the interface between sensory and information processing', in Dawson, G (ed.) *Autism: Nature, Diagnosis and Treatment*, New York: Guilford

Ornitz, E.M., Ritvo, E.R. (1968) *'Perceptual inconstancy in early infantile autism'*, Archives of General Psychiatry, 18, 76-98

Ozonoff, S. (1995) 'Executive function in autism', in Schopler, E., Mesibov, G.B. (eds.) *Diagnosis and Assessment in Autism*, New York: Plenum Press

Park, C.C. (1967) *The Siege: The First Eight Years of an Autistic Child*, Boston: Little, Brown

Patten, B.M. (1973) 'Visually mediated thinking: a report of the case of Albert Einstein', *Journal of Learning Disabilities*, 67, 15-20

Piaget, J. (1952) *The origins of intelligence in children,* New York: International University Press

Rimland, B. (1964) *Infantile Autism: The Syndrome and Its Implications for a Neural Therapy of Behavior,* New York: Appleton-Century-Crofts

Rose, S. (1993) *The Making of Memory: From Molecules to Mind,* London: Bantam Press

Russell, J. (1994) 'Agency and early mental development', in Bermudez, J., Marcel, A.J., Eilan, N. (eds.) *The Body and the Self,* Cambridge Ma MIT Press

Schatzman, M. (1980) *The Story of Ruth,* London: Gerald Duckworth

Sheldrake, R. (1999) *Dogs That Know When Their Owners Are Coming Home,* Hutchinson

Stehli, A. (1991) *Sound of a Miracle,* New York: Avon Books

Walker, N., Cantello J. (eds.) (1994) *You Don't Have Words to Describe What I Experience,* Geneva Centre for Autism, http://www.autism.net/

Waterhouse, S. (2000) *A Positive Approach to Autism,* Jessica Kingsley Publishers: London & Philadelphia

Welling, H. (1994) 'Prime number identification in idiot savants', *Journal of Autism and Developmental Disorders,* 24, 199-207

Wing, L. (1992) *The Triad of Impairments of Social Interaction: an aid to diagnosis,* London: NAS

World Health Organisation (1992) *International Statistical Classification of Diseases and Related Health Problems,* Geneva: WHO

Zeki, S. (1992) 'The visual image in the mind and brain', *Scientific American,* September, 69-76

Key Authors with ASD and Their Works

Blackburn, J. (1997) *Autism? What is it…?* ANI, http://www.planetc.com/

Blackburn, J. (1999) *My Inside View of Autism,* ANI, http://www.planetc.com/

Bovee, J.-P. (Undated) *My Experiences with Autism and How it Relates to Theory of Mind*, Geneva Centre for Autism, http://www.autism.net/infoparent.html

Dekker, M. (Undated) *On Our Terms: Emerging Autistic Culture*, Martin Dekker's files

Gerland, G. (1997) *A Real Person – Life on the Outside*, Translated by J.Tate, London: Souvenir Press

Gerland, G. (1998) 'Now is the time! Autism and psychoanalysis', *Code of Good Practice on Prevention of Violence against Persons with Autism*, Autism-Europe publication, pp. 31-33

Grandin, T. (1992) 'An inside view of autism', in Schopler, E., Mesibov, G.B. (eds.) *High Functioning Individuals with Autism*, New York: Plenum Press

Grandin, T. (1996a) *Thinking in Pictures and Other Reports from My Life with Autism*, Vintage Books. A Division of Random House, Inc. New York

Grandin, T. (1996b) *My Experiences with Visual Thinking Sensory Problems and Communication Difficulties*, Centre for the Study of Autism, http://www.autism.org/

Grandin, T. (1999) *Genius May Be an Abnormality: Educating Students with Asperger's Syndrome or High Functioning Autism*, Autism99 Internet Conference, http://www.autism99.org/

Grandin, T., Scariano, M. (1986) *Emergence Labeled Autistic*, Yunbridge Wells: Costello

Joan and Rich (1999) *What is Autism?* ANT, http://www.staff.uluc.edu/

Joliffe, T., Lakesdown, R., Robinson, C. 'Autism, a personal account', *Communication*, 26(3), 12-19

Kochmeister, S.J. (Undated) *The Continuing Realization of a Dream Too Many Would Choose to Have Deferred Or When the Walls Finally Crumble*, Geneva Centre for Autism, http://www.autism.net/

Lawson, W. (1998) *Life Behind Glass: A personal account of Autism Spectrum Disorder*, Southern Cross University Press

Lawson, W. (1999) *Reflection on Autism and Communication – A Person Account*, Autism99 Internet Conference, http://www.autism99.org/

McKean, Th. (1994) *Soon Will Come the Light*, Future Education, Inc., Arlington, Texas

Morris, B. (1999) *New Light and Insight, on an Old Master, A Glossary for Cygnus Terms,* Autism99 Internet Conference, http://www.autism99.org/

Nony (1993) 'Speculation on light sensitivity', *Our Voice*, 3, 1

O'Neill, J.L. (1999) *Through the Eyes of Aliens: A Book about Autistic People*, Jessica Kingsley Publishers: London and Philadelphia

Rand, B. (Undated) *How To Understand People Who Are Different*, ACCESS, http://access.autistics.org/

Schneider, E. (1999) Discovering My Autism. Apologia Pro Vita Sua (with Apologies to Cardinal Newman), Jessica Kingsley Publishers: London and Philadelphia

Sinclair, J. (1993) 'Don't mourn for us', *Our Voice,* 1(3)

Sinclair, J. (1998) *Is "Cure" a Goal?* Jim Sinclair's Web Page, http://members.xoom.com/

VanDalen, J.G.T. (1995) 'Autism from within: Looking through the eyes of a mildly afflicted autistic person', *Link*, 17, 11-16

White, B.B., White, M.S. (1987) 'Autism from the inside', *Medical Hypotheses,* 24

Willey, L.H. (1999) *Pretending to be Normal: Living with Asperger Syndrome*, Jessica Kingsley Publishers: London and Philadelphia

Williams, D. (1992) *Nobody Nowhere*, London: Doubleday

Williams, D. (1994) *Somebody Somewhere,* London: Doubleday

Williams, D. (1996) *Autism. An Inside-Out Approach*, Jessica Kingsley Publishers: London and Bristol, Pennsylvania

Williams, D. (1998) *Autism and Sensing. The Unlost Instinct*, Jessica Kingsley Publishers: London and Philadelphia

Williams, D. (1999) *Like Colour to the Blind: Soul Searching and Soul Finding,* Jessica Kingsley Publishers: London and Philadelphia

Williams, D. (2000) 'Foreword', in Waterhouse, S. *A Positive Approach to Autism*, Jessica Kingsley Publishers: London and Philadelphia

Appendix 1

QUESTIONNAIRE

SENSORY PROFILE CHECKLIST (SPC)

Name of Child ______________________________ Birthdate ____________

Diagnosed __________________________ When? ___________

Where? ___________________

PURPOSE: This checklist is designed for completion by parents of children who have been diagnosed as "autistic/ASD". The SPC is intended to clarify the sensory experiences of such children and provide sensory profile ("rainbow") in order to identify possible sensory strengths and weaknesses that would be helpful in selecting appropriate methods of teaching and treatment.

INSTRUCTIONS: Please tick the appropriate answer to indicate the statement described as

WT – was true any time in the past; in brackets, specify the age of the child when the statement was true, e.g., (2-5 yrs);

T - true now (if it was true and is true now, tick both answers);

F – false (if the statement is not true);

NS - not sure or don't know

Additional information is welcome: write it near the question, or copy the question number on a blank sheet of paper and add the information there.

Please try to answer all questions.

	WT	T	F	NS
1. Constantly looks at minute particles, picks up smallest pieces of dust, etc.				
2. Dislikes dark and bright lights				
3. Notices every tiny change in the environment				
4. Is frightened by sharp flashes of light, lightning, etc.				
5. Looks down most of the time				
6. Covers or closes eyes at bright lights				
7. Makes sudden but controlled movements				
8. Is attracted to lights				
9. Looks intensely at objects or people				
10. Moves fingers or objects in front of the eyes				
11. Is fascinated with reflections, bright coloured objects				
12. Rocking movements				
13. Runs a hand around the edge of the object				
14. Perimeter hugging				
15. May respond differently (indifference – distress) to the same lights, colours, visual patterns				
16. Does not seem to see if listening to something				
17. Resists to any change				
18. Selects for attention minor aspects of objects in the environment instead of the whole thing, (e.g., a wheel rather than a whole toy car, etc.)				
19. Gets lost easily				

	WT	T	F	NS
20. Does not recognize people in unfamiliar clothes, on photograph				
21. Fears heights, stairs, escalators				
22. Has difficulty catching balls				
23. Appears startled when being approached suddenly				
24. Climbs high into a tree, jumps off tall fences, etc.				
25. Makes compulsive repetitive hand, head or body movements that fluctuate between near and far				
26. Hits/rubs eyes when distressed				
27. Avoids direct eye contact				
28. Is not fooled by optical illusions				
29. Squints or closes eyes in bright light				
30. Gets easily frustrated/tired under fluorescent lights				
31. Gets frustrated with certain colours (Specify:)				
32. Is fascinated with certain coloured and shining objects (Specify:)				
33. Seems to be absorbed (merged) with lights, colours				
34. Seems to know what other people (who are not present) are doing				
35. Response to visual stimuli is delayed, (e.g., fails to close eyes when the light is being suddenly switched on, etc.)				
36. Repetitive blinking and head bobbing				

	WT	T	F	NS
37. Any experiences are perceived as new and unfamiliar, regardless of the number of times the child has experienced the same thing				
38. Sudden outbursts of self-abuse/tantrums or withdrawal in response to a visual stimuli				
39. Appears to be a mindless follower				
40. Feels/acts blind				
41. Ritualistic behaviour				
42. Smells, licks, touches or taps objects				
43. Covers/rubs/blinks, etc. eyes in respond to a sound/touch/smell/taste				
44. Complains about (is frustrated with) the "wrong" colours of letters/numbers, etc. on coloured blocks, etc.				
45. Displays a good visual memory				
46. Reactions are triggered by lights or colours				
47. Easily solves jigsaw puzzles				
48. Remembers the routes and places				
49. Memorizes enormous amounts of information at a glance				
50. Poor at mathematics				
51. Learns nouns first				
52. Has difficulties with adverbs and prepositions				
53. Idiosyncratic patterns in language development (e.g., names one thing to denote the other, etc.)				
54. Covers ears at many sounds				
55. Is a very light sleeper				

	WT	T	F	NS
56. Is frightened by animals				
57. Dislikes thunderstorm, sea, crowds				
58. Dislikes haircut				
59. Avoids sounds and noises				
60. Makes repetitive noises				
61. Bangs objects, doors				
62. Likes vibration				
63. Likes kitchen and bathroom				
64. Likes traffic, crowds				
65. Tears paper, crumples paper in the hand				
66. Is attracted by sounds				
67. Makes rhythmic noises				
68. May respond differently (indifference – distress) to the same sounds, noises				
69. Does not seem to hear if looking at something				
70. Hears a few words instead of the whole sentence				
71. Pronunciation problems				
72. Unable to distinguish between some sounds				
73. Hits ears when distressed				
74. Reacts to the instructions when they are "addressed to the wall"				
75. Gets easily frustrated when trying to do something in a noisy, crowded room				

	WT	T	F	NS
76. Gets frustrated with certain sounds (Specify:)				
77. Tries to destroy/break objects producing sounds (clock, telephone, musical toy, etc.)				
78. Is fascinated with certain sounds (Specify:)				
79. Seems to be absorbed (merged) with sounds				
80. Seems to be able 'to read' thoughts, feelings, etc. of others				
81. Complains about 'non-existent' conversations, sounds				
82. Response to questions, instructions is delayed				
83. Echolalia in monotonous, high-pitched, parrotlike voice				
84. Sudden outbursts of self-abuse/tantrums or withdrawal in response to auditory stimuli				
85. Surprises with knowing "unknown" information				
86. Feels/acts deaf				
87. Looks for the source of the sound				
88. Covers/hits ears in response to lights, colours/touch, texture/smell/taste				
89. Complains about (is frustrated) with a sound in response to colours/textures/touch/scent/flavour				
90. Displays a good auditory memory (for nursery rhymes, songs, etc.)				
91. Reactions are triggered by sounds/words				
92. Uses idiosyncratic routinised responses				
93. Cannot keep track of conversation				

	WT	T	F	NS
94 Uses songs, commercials, etc. to respond				
95. Composes musical pieces, songs				
96. Resists being touched				
97. Cannot tolerate new clothes				
98. Avoids wearing shoes				
99. Overreacts to heat/cold/pain				
100. Avoids getting messy				
101. Dislikes food of certain textures				
102. Moves away from people				
103. Likes pressure, tight clothing				
104. Prone to self-injures				
105. Low reaction to pain, temperature				
106. Places the body in strange positions				
107. Unaware of his own body sensations (e.g., does not feel hunger, etc.)				
108. May respond differently to the same clothes, touch				
109. Does not seem to feel being touched if looking at/listening to or talking to somebody				
110. Complains about parts of the clothes				
111. Enjoys swings, merry-go-rounds				
112. Spins, runs round and round				
113. Hits oneself when distressed				
114. Can tolerate only "instrumental" (not "social") touch				

	WT	T	F	NS
115. Unable to distinguish between tactile stimuli of different intensity (e.g., light and rough touch)				
116. Cannot tolerate certain textures (Specify:)				
117. Is fascinated with certain textures (Specify:)				
118. Seems to be absorbed (merged) with certain textures				
119. Seems to feel pain of others				
120. Complains about 'non-existent' physical experiences (e.g., "I am flying", etc.)				
121. Sudden outbursts of self-abuse/tantrums or withdrawal in response to tactile stimuli				
122. Sometimes does not react to any tactile stimuli				
123. Feels/acts numb				
124 Taps objects				
125. Complains about (is frustrated with) feeling colours, sounds, etc., when being touched				
126. Complains about (is frustrated with) feeling being touched when being looked at				
127. Complains about (is frustrated with) backache, etc./heat/cold in colourful/noisy/crowded places				
128. Involuntary movements/postures of the body in response to a visual/auditory stimulus/smell/taste				
129. Displays a good tactile memory				
130. Reactions are triggered by textures				
131. Toiletting problems				

	WT	T	F	NS
132. Runs from smells				
133. Wears the same clothes				
134. Avoids people				
135. Smells self, people, objects, etc.				
136. Smears/plays with feces				
137. Seeks strong odours				
138. Bedwetting				
139. May respond differently (indifference – distress) to the same smells				
140. Does not seem to feel smell when looking/listening, etc.				
141. Complains about smells of some pieces of food while ignoring the rest				
142. Hits nose when distressed				
143. Avoids direct smell (e.g., leaves the kitchen when one is cooking)				
144. Unable to distinguish between strong and weak odours				
145. Cannot tolerate certain smells (Specify:)				
146. Is fascinated with some smells (Specify:)				
147. Seems to be absorbed (merged) with smells				
148. Complains/talks about 'non-existent' smells				
149. Response to smells is delayed				

	WT	T	F	NS
150. Sudden outbursts of self-abuse/tantrums or withdrawal in response to smells				
151. Sometimes does not react to any smell				
152. Has difficulty in interpreting smells				
153. Inspects food before eating				
154. Covers/rubs/hits, etc. nose in response to a visual/auditory stimulus/touch/taste				
155. Complains about (is frustrated with) the smell in response to a visual/ auditory stimulus/touch/taste				
156. Displays a good memory for smells				
157. Reactions are triggered by smells				
158. Complains about smells while reading, talking, etc.				
159. Poor eater				
160. Uses the tip of the tongue for tasting				
161. Gags/vomits easily				
162. Craves certain foods				
163. Eats anything (Pica)				
164. Mouths and licks objects				
165 Eats mixed food (e.g. sweet and sour)				
166. Regurgitates				
167. May respond differently (indifference – distress) to the same food				
168. Does not feel any taste while eating something and looking at/listening to something				
169. Complains about the food he used to like				

	WT	T	F	NS
170. Seems confused about certain foods				
171. Very careful eater				
172. Unable to distinguish between strong and weak tastes				
173. Cannot tolerate certain food (Specify:)				
174. Is fascinated with certain tastes				
175. Seems to be absorbed (merged) with certain food				
176. Complains/talks about 'non-existent' taste in his mouth				
177. Response to tastes is delayed				
178. Sudden outbursts of self-abuse/tantrums or withdrawal in response to taste				
179. Sometimes does not react to any taste				
180. Has difficulty in interpreting tastes				
181. Makes swallowing movements in response to a visual/auditory stimulus/smell/touch				
182. Complains about (is frustrated with) some tastes in response to a visual/ auditory stimulus/touch/smell				
183. Displays a good memory for tastes				
184. Reactions are triggered by certain food				
185. Complains about feeling tastes while reading, talking, etc.				

Appendix 2

KEY FOR DECODING THE QUESTIONNAIRE

This key will aid you in completing the chart and rainbow.

If you have ticked the 'True' box for a question in the pre-sensory profile checklist then you will need to colour in the corresponding box in the chart. For example, if you have answered question 15 as 'True' then you colour in box 2 in the V column.

Some questions in the profile relate to the same box in the chart. For example, if you have answered 'True' to either question 76 or 77, colour in the box 8 in the H column.

Once you have completed the chart count the number of coloured boxes in the corresponding section. Colour in the same number of boxes in the corresponding section of the rainbow. For example, if you have coloured in 10 boxes in the V column, then colour in 10 boxes of the V section of the rainbow.

1-7 (hyper) 8-14 (hypo)	V 1	54-60 61-67	H 1	96-102 103-107	Tc 1
15	V 2	68	H 2	108	Tc 2
16	V 3	69	H 3	109	Tc 3
17-20	V 4	70	H 4	110	Tc 4
21-26	V 5	71-73	H 5	111-113	Tc 5, V 5
27	V 6	74	H 6	114	Tc 6
28	V 7	75	H 7	115	Tc 7
29-31	V 8	76-77	H 8	116	Tc 8
32	V 9	78	H 9	117	Tc 9
33	V 10	79-80	H 10	118-119	Tc 10
34	V 11	81	H 11	120	Tc 11
35-36	V 12	82-83	H 12	121	Tc 13
37	V 12 H 12 Tc 12	84	H 13	122	Tc 14
38	V 13	85	H 14 V 14	123	Tc 15
39	V 14, H 14	86	H 15	124	Tc 16
40	V 15	87	H 16	125-128	Tc 17
41	V 15, H 15, Tc 15	88-89	H 17	129	Tc 18
42	V 16	90	H 18	130	Tc 19
42-44	V 17	91-94	H 19		
45	V 18	95	H 20		
46	V 19				
47-53	V 20				

131-134 (hyper) 135-138 (hypo)	S 1	159-162 163-166	T1
139	S 2	167	T 2
140	S 3	168	T 3
141	S 4	169	T 4
142	S 5	170	T 5
143	S 6	171	T 6
144	S 7	172	T 7
145	S 8	173	T 8
146	S 9	174	T 9
147	S 10	175	T 10
148	S 11	176	T 11
149	S 12	177	T 12
150	S 13	178	T 13
151	S 14	179	T 14
152	S 15	180	T 15
153	S 16, T 16	181-182	T 17
154-155	S 17	183	T 18
156	S 18	184	T 19
157	S 19	185	T 20
158	S 20		

Photocopiable Chart and Rainbow

	V	H	Tc	T	S
1					
2					
3					
4					
5					
6					
7					
8					
9					
10					
11					
12					
13					
14					
15					
16					
17					
18					
19					
20					

Key

V = red
H = orange
Tc = yellow
T = green
S = blue

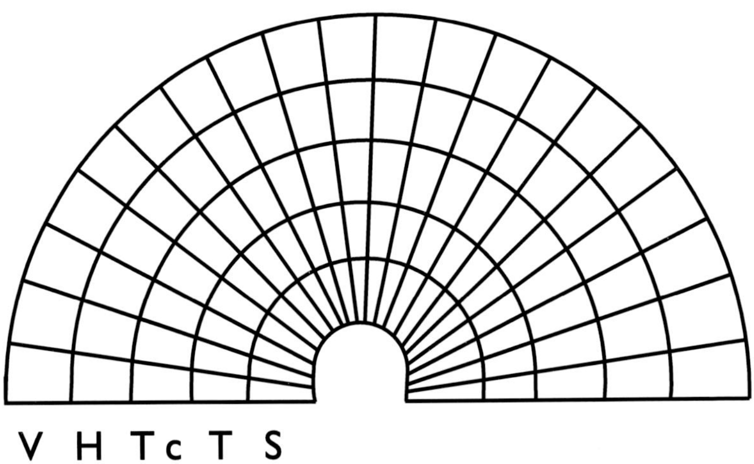